A Practical Guide to

Chemical Peels, Microdermabrasion, & Topical Products

A Practical Guide to

Chemical Peels, Microdermabrasion, & Topical Products

Series Editor
Rebecca Small, MD, FAAFP

Assistant Clinical Professor
Department of Family and Community Medicine
University of California, San Francisco, CA

Director, Medical Aesthetics Training
Natividad Medical Center
Family Medicine Residency Program—UCSF Affiliate
Salinas, CA

Associate Editors
Dalano Hoang, DC

Clinic Director
Monterey Bay Laser Aesthetics
Capitola, CA

Jennifer Linder, MD, FAAD

Assistant Clinical Professor
Department of Dermatology
University of California, San Francisco

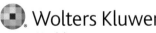
Wolters Kluwer | Lippincott Williams & Wilkins
Health

Philadelphia • Baltimore • New York • London
Buenos Aires • Hong Kong • Sydney • Tokyo

Senior Acquisitions Editor: Sonya Seigafuse
Senior Product Manager: Kerry Barrett
Vendor Manager: Bridgett Dougherty
Senior Manufacturing Manager: Benjamin Rivera
Senior Marketing Manager: Kim Schonberger
Illustrator: Liana Bauman
Creative Director: Doug Smock
Production Service: Aptara, Inc.

Library of Congress Cataloging-in-Publication Data
ISBN-13: 978-1-60913-151-7
ISBN-10: 1-60913-151-7

Care has been taken to confirm the accuracy of the information presented and to describe generally accepted practices. However, the authors, editors, and publisher are not responsible for errors or omissions or for any consequences from application of the information in this book and make no warranty, expressed or implied, with respect to the currency, completeness, or accuracy of the contents of the publication. Application of the information in a particular situation remains the professional responsibility of the practitioner.

The authors, editors, and publisher have exerted every effort to ensure that drug selection and dosage set forth in this text are in accordance with current recommendations and practice at the time of publication. However, in view of ongoing research, changes in government regulations, and the constant flow of information relating to drug therapy and drug reactions, the reader is urged to check the package insert for each drug for any change in indications and dosage and for added warnings and precautions. This is particularly important when the recommended agent is a new or infrequently employed drug.

Some drugs and medical devices presented in the publication have Food and Drug Administration (FDA) clearance for limited use in restricted research settings. It is the responsibility of the health care provider to ascertain the FDA status of each drug or device planned for use in their clinical practice.

To purchase additional copies of this book, call our customer service department at (800) 638-3030 or fax orders to (301) 223-2320. International customers should call (301) 223-2300.

Visit Lippincott Williams & Wilkins on the Internet: at LWW.com. Lippincott Williams & Wilkins customer service representatives are available from 8:30 am to 6 pm, EST.

19 18 17 16 15 14 13 12 11

As a lecturer, editor, author, and medical reviewer, I have had ample opportunity to evaluate many speakers as well as extensive medical literature. After reviewing this series of books on cosmetic procedures by Rebecca Small, MD, I have concluded that it has to be one of the best and most detailed, yet practical presentation of the topics that I have ever encountered. As a physician whose practice is limited solely to providing office procedures, I see great value in these texts for clinicians and the patients they serve.

The goal of medical care is to make patients feel better and to help them experience an improved quality of life that extends for an optimal, productive period. Interventions may be directed at the emotional/psychiatric, medical/physical, or self-image areas.

For many physicians, performing medical procedures provides excitement in the practice of medicine. The ability to see what has been accomplished in a concrete way provides the positive feedback we all seek in providing care. Sometimes, it involves removing a tumor. At other times, it may be performing a screening procedure to be sure no disease is present. Maybe it is making patients feel better about their appearance. For whatever reason, the "hands on" practice of medicine is more rewarding for some practitioners.

In the late 1980s and early 1990s, there was resurgence in the interest of performing procedures in primary care. It did not involve hospital procedures but rather those that could be performed in the office. Coincidentally, patients also became interested in less invasive procedures such as laparoscopic cholecystectomy, endometrial ablation, and more. The desire for plastic surgery "extreme makeovers" waned, as technology was developed to provide a gentle, more kind approach to "rejuvenation." Baby boomers were increasing in numbers and wanted to maintain their youthful appearance. This not only improved self-image but it also helped when competing with a younger generation both socially and in the workplace.

These forces then of technological advances, provider interest, and patient desires have led to a huge increase in and demand for "minimally invasive procedures" that has extended to all of medicine. Plastic surgery and aesthetic procedures have indeed been affected by this movement. There have been many new procedures developed in just the last 10–15 years along with constant updates and improvements. As patient demand has soared for these new treatments, physicians have found that there is a whole new world of procedures they need to incorporate into their practice if they are going to provide the latest in aesthetic services.

Rebecca Small, MD, the editor and author of this series of books on cosmetic procedures, has been at the forefront of the aesthetic procedures movement. She has written extensively and conducted numerous workshops to help others learn the latest techniques. She has the practical experience to know just what the physician needs to develop a practice and provides "the latest and the best" in these books. Using her knowledge of the field, she has selected the topics wisely to include

- A Practical Guide to: Botulinum Toxin Procedures
- A Practical Guide to: Dermal Filler Procedures
- A Practical Guide to: Chemical Peels, Microdermabrasion and Topical Products
- A Practical Guide to: Cosmetic Laser Procedures

Dr. Small does not just provide a cursory, quick review of these subjects. Rather, they are an in-depth practical guide to performing these procedures. The emphasis here should be on "practical" and "in-depth." There is no extra esoteric waste of words, yet every procedure is explained in a clear, concise, useful format that allows practitioners of all levels of experience to learn and gain from reading these texts.

The basic outline of these books consists of the pertinent anatomy, the specific indications and contraindications, specific how-to diagrams and explanations on performing the procedures, complications and how to deal with them, tables with comparisons and amounts of materials needed, before and after patient instructions as well as consent forms (an immense time-saving feature), sample procedure notes, and a list of supply sources. An extensive updated bibliography is provided in each text for further reading. Photos are abundant depicting the performance of the procedures as well as before and after results. These comprehensive texts are clearly written for the practitioner who wants to "learn everything" about the topics covered. Patients definitely desire these procedures and Dr. Small has provided the information to meet the physician demand to learn them.

For those interested in aesthetic procedures, these books will be a godsend. Even for those not so interested in performing the procedures described, the reading is easy and interesting and will update the readers on what is currently available so that they might better advise their patients.

Dr. Small has truly written a one-of-a-kind series of books on Cosmetic Procedures. It is my prediction that it will be received very well and be most appreciated by all who make use of it.

John L. Pfenninger, MD, FAAFP
Founder and President, The Medical Procedures Center
PC Founder and Senior Consultant, The National Procedures Institute
Clinical Professor of Family Medicine, Michigan State College
of Human Medicine

Following publication of the article "Aesthetic Procedures in Office Practice", I have received numerous inquiries and requests for aesthetic training from providers and residents. The common thread of these inquiries has been a need for educational resources and quality training in aesthetic procedures that can be readily incorporated into office practice.

As the trend in aesthetic medicine shifts away from radical surgeries toward procedures that offer more subtle enhancements, the number of minimally invasive aesthetic procedures performed continues to grow. These procedures (which include chemical peels, microdermabrasion, topical products, dermal filler and botulinum toxin injections, lasers, and light-based technologies) have become the primary modalities for treatment of facial aging and skin rejuvenation. This cosmetic procedures book series is designed to be a truly practical guide for physicians, physician assistants, nurse practitioners, residents in training, and other healthcare providers interested in aesthetics. It is not comprehensive, but is inclusive of current minimally invasive aesthetic procedures that can be readily incorporated into office practice, that directly benefit our patients and reliably achieve good outcomes with a low incidence of side-effects.

The goal of this book on skin care procedures and topical products, the third in the cosmetic practical guide series, is to provide step-by-step instructions for in-office exfoliation treatments and daily home skin care regimens to treat photoaged skin. The Introduction serves as a foundation and provides basic aesthetic medicine concepts essential to successfully performing aesthetic procedures. Relevant anatomy is reviewed, including the target regions and areas to be avoided, to help providers perform procedures more effectively and minimize complications. Each section is dedicated to a skin care procedure or topical product regimen and each chemical peel chapter focuses on application techniques for a specific peel. There are accompanying instructional videos demonstrating the procedures. While the treatments in this book have been chosen based on their low incidence of complications, suggestions for management of complications as well as the most commonly encountered issues seen in follow-up visits are discussed. Also included are up-to-date suggestions for treatment of other common aesthetic skin complaints including hyperpigmentation, rosacea and acne. The experienced provider may appreciate suggestions for combining aesthetic treatments to maximize outcomes, current product developments and reimbursement recommendations.

When getting started with exfoliation procedures, providers are encouraged to begin with the basic superficial chemical peels and conservative microdermabrasion settings, then progress to more aggressive peels and higher settings as knowledge and skill are acquired. Enhanced results, whether treating photoaged skin or other aesthetic skin conditions, can be achieved by combining chemical peels, microdermabrasion and topical products using the methods described in this practical guide. In addition, these therapies can also be safely combined with laser or light-based procedures and dermal filler and botulinum toxin injections to address more advanced aging changes.

This book is intended to serve as a guide and not a replacement for experience. When learning aesthetic procedural skills, a formal training course is recommended, as well as preceptorship with an experienced provider.

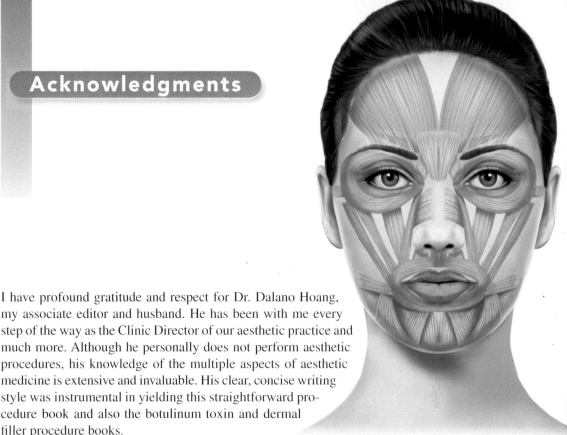

Acknowledgments

I have profound gratitude and respect for Dr. Dalano Hoang, my associate editor and husband. He has been with me every step of the way as the Clinic Director of our aesthetic practice and much more. Although he personally does not perform aesthetic procedures, his knowledge of the multiple aspects of aesthetic medicine is extensive and invaluable. His clear, concise writing style was instrumental in yielding this straightforward procedure book and also the botulinum toxin and dermal filler procedure books.

I would also like to thank Dr. Jennifer Linder, my other associate editor. Her knowledge and expertise on skin care procedures and products greatly contributed to this book.

Special thanks goes to Dr. John L. Pfenninger and Dr. E.J. Mayeaux, who have inspired and supported me, and taught me much about educating and writing.

The University of California San Francisco and the Natividad Medical Center family medicine residents deserve special recognition. Their interest and enthusiasm for aesthetic procedures led me to develop the first family medicine aesthetics training curriculum in 2008. Special recognition is also due to the primary care providers who participated in my aesthetic courses at the American Academy of Family Practice national conferences over the years. Their questions and input further solidified the need for this practical guide series.

I am indebted to my Capitola office staff for their ongoing logistical and administrative support, especially Tiffany Sorensen. Her practical knowledge and expertise as a clinical aesthetician are greatly appreciated.

Special acknowledgements are due to those at Wolters Kluwer Health who made this book series possible, in particular, Sonya Seigafuse, Doug Smock, Nicole Dernoski, Freddie Patane, as well as Indu Jawwad and Jenny Ceccotti at Aptara. It has been a pleasure working with Liana Bauman, the gifted artist who created all of the illustrations for these books.

Finally, I would like to dedicate this third book in the series to my son, Kaidan Hoang, for the unending hugs and kisses that greeted me no matter how late I got home from working on this project.

Contents

   Procedure videos can be found on the book's website.

Anatomy

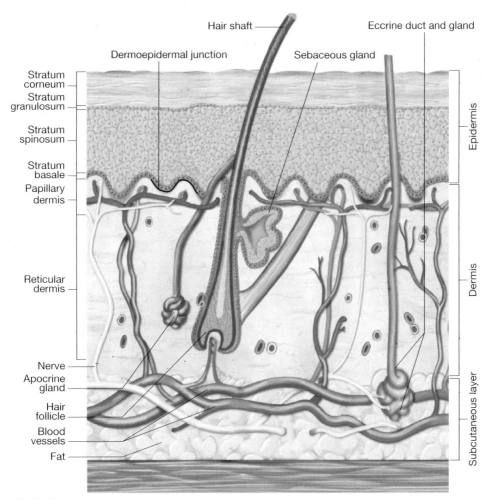

FIGURE 1 ● Skin anatomy

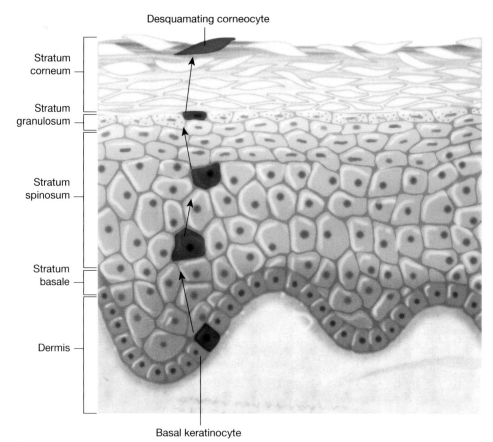

Desquamating corneocyte

Stratum corneum

Stratum granulosum

Stratum spinosum

Stratum basale

Dermis

Basal keratinocyte

FIGURE 2 ● Epidermis

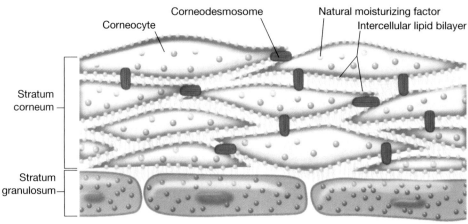

Corneocyte

Corneodesmosome

Natural moisturizing factor
Intercellular lipid bilayer

Stratum corneum

Stratum granulosum

FIGURE 3 ● Stratum corneum

Depth of Resurfacing

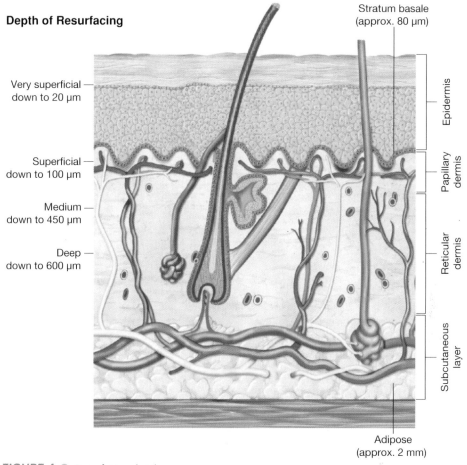

FIGURE 4 ● Resurfacing depths

Introduction and Foundation Concepts

Office-based exfoliation procedures such as chemical peels and microdermabrasion, and topical products designed for daily use can be incorporated into any type of medical practice to help patients attain healthy skin and enhance appearance. They are also commonly used to support and augment the results of other aesthetic procedures such as laser, intense-pulsed light and injectable treatments. Getting started in this area of medicine can be a daunting task given the plethora of available treatment options and information, much of which is unsubstantiated. This practical guide distills clinically relevant information, presenting it in a simple format, for evaluation and management of common dermatologic conditions and cosmetic complaints, with a focus on sun damaged skin. Each of the treatments discussed can stand-alone; however, combining them appropriately can improve outcomes. This integrated approach is also highly modifiable and allows providers to tailor therapies to meet patient's specific needs. Management strategies for hyperpigmentation, facial erythema such as rosacea and sensitive skin, and acne are also discussed, along with suggestions for combining skin care with other aesthetic procedures such as laser and injectable treatments.

Skin Aging

The visible signs of aging are caused by a combination of physiologic (intrinsic) and environmental (extrinsic) factors. Over-exposure to ultraviolet (UV) radiation is one of the main factors responsible for cutaneous damage and these effects are commonly referred to as sun damage, photoaging, actinic damage and UV-induced aging. Other extrinsic aging factors include smoking, diet, sleep habits, and alcohol consumption. Photoaging can present with one or more of the following clinical findings (Fig. 1 and figures listed below):

- Textural changes
  - Wrinkles (Fig. 2)
  - Dilated pores (Fig. 3)
  - Dry and rough skin
  - Solar elastosis (Fig. 4)
- Sagging and laxity (Fig. 5)
- Pigmentary changes
  - Hyperpigmentation: lentigines (Figs. 4, 6, and 10), darkened freckles (Fig. 7), mottled pigmentation (Figs. 8 and 9)
  - Poikiloderma of Civatte (Fig. 11)
  - Hypopigmentation (Fig. 12)
  - Sallow discoloration (Fig. 4)
- Vascular changes
  - Telangiectasias (Fig. 13) and erythema

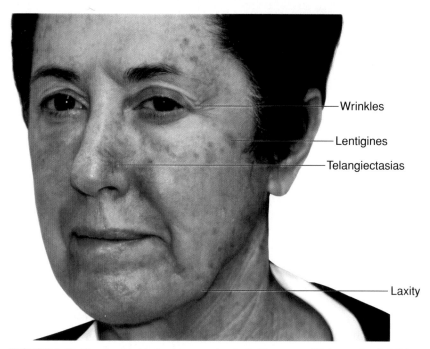

Wrinkles

Lentigines

Telangiectasias

Laxity

FIGURE 1 ● Photoaged skin (computer enhanced). (Courtesy of Rebecca Small, MD)

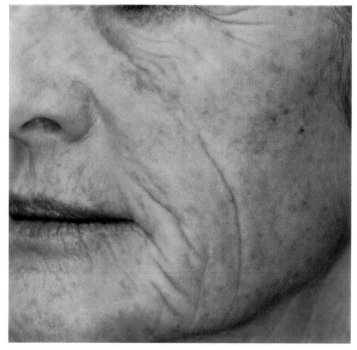

FIGURE 2 ● Wrinkles. (Courtesy of Rebecca Small, MD)

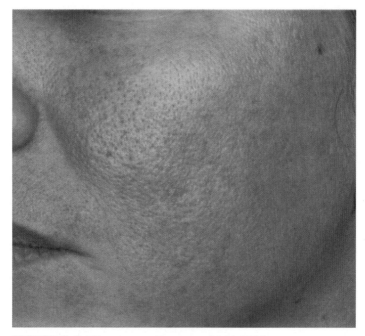

FIGURE 3 ● Dilated pores. (Courtesy of PCA SKIN)

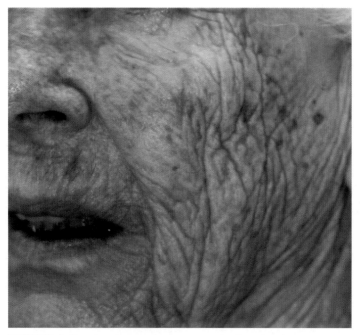

FIGURE 4 ● Solar elastosis, lentigines, and sallow discoloration. (Courtesy of Rebecca Small, MD)

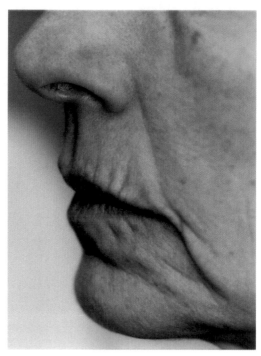

FIGURE 5 ● Sagging and laxity. (Courtesy of Rebecca Small, MD)

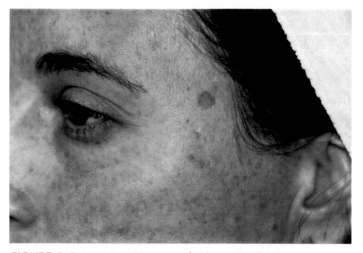

FIGURE 6 ● Lentigines (Courtesy of Rebecca Small, MD)

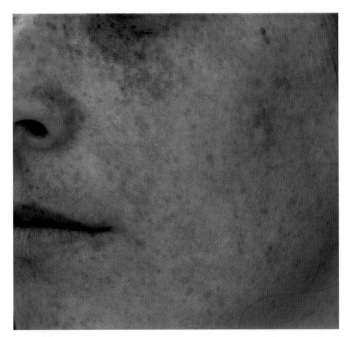

FIGURE 7 ● Darkened freckles. (Courtesy of Rebecca Small, MD)

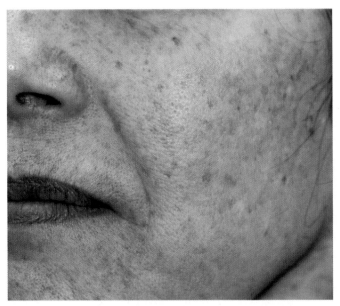

FIGURE 8 ● Mottled pigmentation on the face. (Courtesy of Rebecca Small, MD)

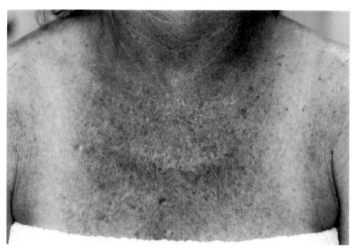

FIGURE 9 ● Mottled pigmentation on the chest. (Courtesy of Rebecca Small, MD)

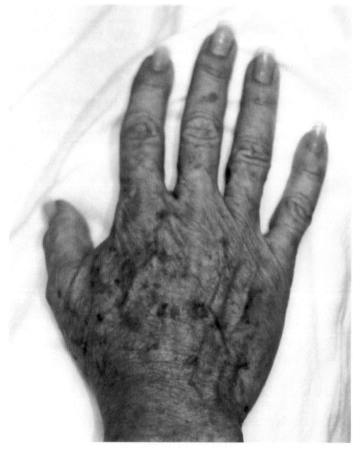

FIGURE 10 ● Lentigines, seborrheic keratoses, and thinning skin. (Courtesy of Rebecca Small, MD)

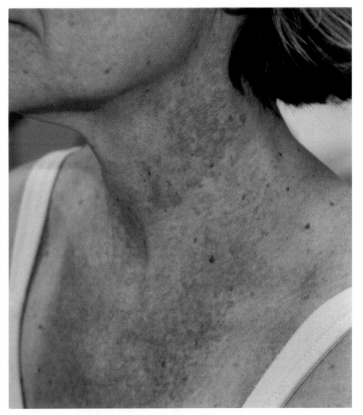

FIGURE 11 ● Poikiloderma of Civatte. (Courtesy of Rebecca Small, MD)

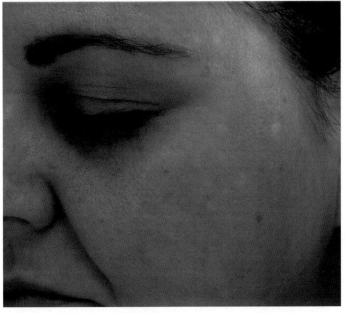

FIGURE 12 ● Hypopigmentation. (Courtesy of Jennifer Linder, MD)

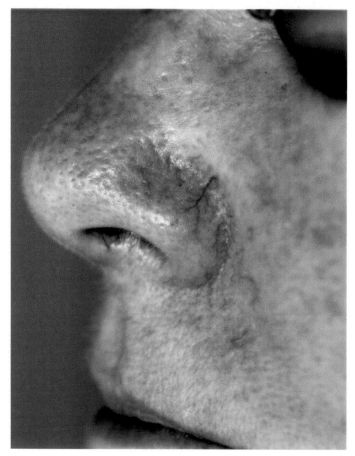

FIGURE 13 ● Telangiectasias. (Courtesy of Rebecca Small, MD)

- Degenerative changes
  - Benign (seborrheic keratoses [Figs. 10 and 14], sebaceous hyperplasia [Fig. 15], cherry angiomas [Fig. 16])
  - Preneoplastic and neoplastic (actinic keratoses, basal and squamous cell cancers, and melanomas)

Skin Anatomy

The skin is divided into 3 layers: the epidermis, dermis, and subcutaneous layer (see Anatomy section, Fig. 1). The structure and function of the different skin layers and components are summarized in Appendix 1.

The **epidermis** is the top layer of the skin and is composed of four cell types: keratinocytes, melanocytes, Langerhans cells, and Merkel cells. The epidermis is further divided into the outermost non-living layer, the stratum corneum, and the living cellular layers of the stratum granulosum, stratum spinosum, and stratum basale (see Anatomy section, Fig. 2).

The stratum corneum is composed of corneocytes (non-living keratinocytes) and lipids, and is referred to as the epidermal barrier. It functions as an evaporative

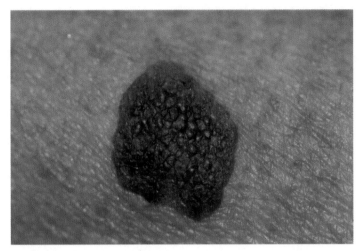

FIGURE 14 ● Seborrheic keratosis. (Courtesy of Rebecca Small, MD)

barrier maintaining skin hydration and suppleness, and as a protective physical barrier against microbes, trauma, irritants, and ultraviolet light. Corneocytes contain the skin's natural moisturizing factor (NMF) which maintains hydration of the stratum corneum. Corneocytes are adhered to one another by corneodesmosomes. A lipid bilayer surrounds the corneocytes which is comprised of 2 layers of phospholipids that have hydrophilic heads and two hydrophobic tails (see Anatomy section, Fig. 3). The epidermis requires continual renewal to maintain its integrity and function effectively. In young healthy skin, it takes approximately 1 month for keratinocytes to migrate from the living basal layer of the epidermis to the stratum corneum surface and desquamate during the epidermal renewal process. Figure 2 in the Anatomy section shows the structure of the epidermis with the keratinocyte maturation process highlighted.

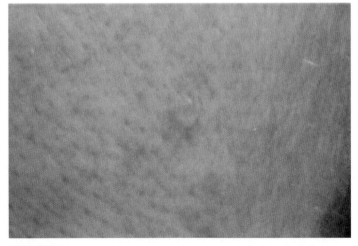

FIGURE 15 ● Sebaceous hyperplasia. (Courtesy of Jennifer Linder, MD)

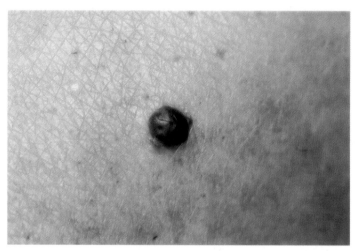

FIGURE 16 ● Cherry angioma. (Courtesy of Rebecca Small, MD)

Melanin pigment, which determines skin color and causes hyperpigmentation, is primarily concentrated within the epidermis, and in some conditions is found in the dermis (e.g., some forms of melasma). There are two types of melanin pigment: pheomelanin and eumelanin. Pheomelanin is yellow to red in color and is found in light skin. Eumelanin is brown to black in color and is the predominant type of melanin in darker skin. Melanin synthesis (melanogenesis) occurs within melanocytes in the basal layer of the epidermis. The key regulatory step is the initial enzymatic conversion of tyrosine to melanin by tyrosinase. Melanin is packaged into melanosomes, intracellular organelles within the melanocyte, which are then distributed to surrounding epidermal keratinocytes (Fig. 17). Melanin has a protective physiologic role in the skin to shield keratinocyte nuclei by absorbing harmful UV radiation; and eumelanin has the greatest UV absorption capabilities. When skin is exposed to UV radiation, melanin synthesis is upregulated which is clinically apparent as skin darkening or tanned skin. The number of melanocytes is similar for both light and dark skin types; however, the quantity and distribution of melanin within the epidermis differ. Light skin has less melanin per square centimeter and smaller melanosomes that are closely aggregated in membrane-bound clusters. Dark skin has more melanin and larger melanosomes that are distributed singly (Fig. 18).

The **dermis** lies beneath the epidermis and is divided into the more superficial papillary dermis and deeper reticular dermis (see Anatomy section, Fig. 1). The main cell type in the dermis is the fibroblast, which is abundant in the papillary dermis and sparse in the reticular dermis. Fibroblasts synthesize most components of the dermal extracellular matrix (ECM), which includes structural proteins such as collagen and elastin, glycosaminoglycans such as hyaluronic acid, and adhesive proteins such as fibronectin and laminins.

Below the dermis and above the underlying muscle is the **subcutaneous layer** or superficial fascia. This layer is composed of both fatty and fibrous components.

Histology of Skin Aging

Photoaged skin has slower, disorganized keratinocyte maturation and increased cellular adhesion relative to healthy, young skin. These factors reduce desquamation and

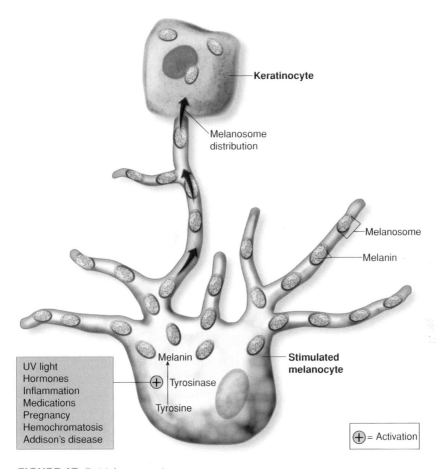

FIGURE 17 ● Melanogenesis.

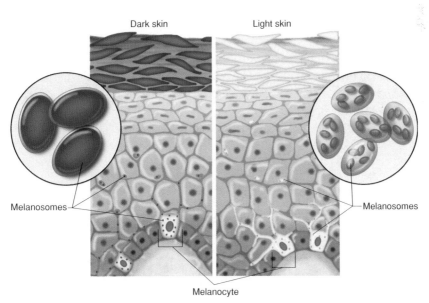

FIGURE 18 ● Dark and light skin characteristics.

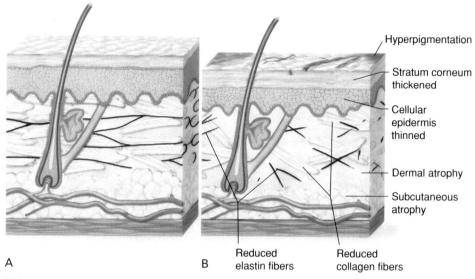

Hyperpigmentation

Stratum corneum thickened

Cellular epidermis thinned

Dermal atrophy

Subcutaneous atrophy

A   B   Reduced   Reduced
                                                      elastin fibers   collagen fibers

FIGURE 19 ● Young (A) and photoaged (B) skin.

result in a rough and thickened stratum corneum which has impaired barrier function. The stratum corneum also has poor light reflectance which is evident as dullness or a sallow (yellow-gray) discoloration. Water escapes more freely from the skin causing dehydration, which can be measured as increased transepidermal water loss (TEWL). The disrupted epidermal barrier also allows for increased irritant penetration which can be associated with skin sensitivity and erythema. Photoaged skin also demonstrates pigmentary changes due to overactive melanocytes and disorganized melanin deposition in the epidermis. Regions with excess melanin are evident as hyperpigmentation and regions with melanin deficits appear as hypopigmentation.

In the dermis, chronic UV exposure has many damaging effects on the ECM. Structural proteins such as collagen are degraded due to upregulation of enzymes (e.g., matrix metalloproteinases), and weakened due to crosslinkage. This accelerated collagen degradation combined with reduced collagen synthesis that occurs over time, contribute to formation of fine lines and wrinkles. In certain cases of advanced photoaging, solar elastosis occurs which consists of tangled masses of damaged elastin protein in the dermis; seen clinically as coarse wrinkling, sallow discoloration, and skin thickening. Abnormal dilation of dermal blood vessels is also common, leading to visible facial erythema and telangiectasias. Figure 19 illustrates histologic changes of photoaged skin.

Ethnic Skin Considerations

In addition to differences in coloration, other histologic and pathophysiologic differences exist between light and dark skin. The stratum corneum is thicker in dark skin, which may contribute to skin conditions exacerbated by compaction, such as acne. The dermis also tends to be thicker in dark skin. Dermal blood vessels are more prominent and dilated, suggesting an exaggerated inflammatory response, which may contribute to increased susceptibility to hyperpigmentation.

Exfoliation Procedures

Regular exfoliation with procedures such as chemical peels and microdermabrasion, combined with daily home skin care products, improves overall skin function and appearance, and effectively treats photodamaged skin. These exfoliation procedures, also referred to as superficial skin resurfacing treatments, remove the outer skin layers by chemical or mechanical methods, respectively. Their effects on skin are based on the principles of wound healing whereby, controlled wounding of the epidermis with removal of superficial skin layers stimulates cell renewal and generates a healthier epidermis and dermis.

The skin's natural cell turnover process is a complex series of steps that ultimately leads to the shedding of cornified dead skin cells. This process can be easily disrupted with aging, skin diseases, and environmental insults. Improper desquamation leads to a dull complexion as well as rough, dry skin and is a key contributor to many common skin concerns.

Regardless of the exfoliation method used the effects are similar, to regulate the skin's natural epidermal renewal process, stimulate production of ECM components such as collagen and glycosaminoglycans, even melanin distribution, and improve epidermal barrier function. Histologic changes observed in the skin after a series of exfoliation treatments include a thinned, smoother stratum corneum, increased dermal thickness with enhanced production of new collagen and elastin, and increased skin hydration. Visible clinical improvements may be seen in rough skin texture, fine lines, pore size, superficial acne scars, acne, and hyperpigmentation.

Chemical Peels

Chemical peels are primarily acids that are applied topically to remove the outer layers of skin. Chemical peels can be classified based on their depth of skin penetration as follows: superficial, medium, and deep (see Anatomy section, Fig. 4). This book focuses on superficial peels which partially or fully remove the stratum corneum and may penetrate the epidermis. Examples of different types of chemical peels are given in the table below. More detailed information is provided in the Introduction and Foundation Concepts of the Chemical Peels section, with specific techniques for application in the individual chapters.

Chemical Peel Types	Examples of Superficial Peeling Agents
Alpha hydroxy acids	Lactic acid, glycolic acid
Beta hydroxy acids	Salicylic acid
Trichloroacetic acid	Trichloroacetic acid up to 20%
Blended peels: self-neutralizing	Jessner's peel (lactic acid/salicylic acid/resorcinol), salicylic acid/mandelic acid
Blended peels: requiring neutralization	Glycolic acid/any other peel
Retinoids	Retinoic acid, retinol

Chemical peel products for use in the office, also known as back bar products, can be purchased from chemical peel companies or from clinical skin care companies. Some companies manufacture or distribute peels and they may have more competitive pricing. Clinical skin care companies usually offer additional support with training and education, and may have topical skin care product lines that complement their chemical peels. Chemical peel suppliers are listed in Appendix 8, Chemical Peel and Topical Product Supply Sources.

Microdermabrasion

Microdermabrasion (MDA) is a mechanical exfoliation procedure for superficial skin resurfacing. Equipment for MDA typically consists of a closed-loop vacuum that draws the skin up to an abrasive element at the handpiece, such as a diamond-tipped pad or aerosolized particles. The abrasive element is passed across the skin to superficially abrade the skin's surface. Surface debris is aspirated and collected for disposal after treatment. The stratum corneum is fully removed with two passes of most MDA devices which achieves a resurfacing depth comparable to superficial chemical peels. Additional information is provided in the Microdermabrasion section of this book. Microdermabrasion suppliers are listed in Appendix 7.

Topical Skin Care Products

Topical skin care products can be used to improve the appearance of and promote healthy skin in any patient. They range in strength from prescription or over-the-counter (OTC) drugs that affect the structure and function of skin, to cosmetic products that alter the appearance of skin. Cosmeceuticals lie within this spectrum of product types, and deliver perceptible skin benefits.

The following section focuses on products that are designed to cleanse, treat, and protect photoaged skin, referred to as the Topical Product Regimen for Photoaged Skin. An overview and rationale for the Regimen is provided below with greater detail discussed in the Topical Skin Care Products section. These rejuvenation products, consisting primarily of cosmeceuticals, have also been selected on the basis of their compatibility with superficial chemical peels and/or MDA treatments as combination therapy enhances results. Many alternative selections of topical products are equally appropriate. When treating other skin conditions such as facial erythema in patients with rosacea and sensitive skin, acne, or hyperpigmentation, the Topical Product Regimen can be modified to address each specific skin condition. Recommendations for regimens to address these specific conditions are discussed in the Topical Skin Care Product section.

Topical Product Regimen for Photoaged Skin

1. **Gentle facial cleanser**
   The purpose of a cleanser is to remove dirt, oil, makeup, and other debris from the skin and allow other products to work more efficiently. This is the first step in any daily skin care regimen and is performed prior to application of topical treatment products. An ideal cleanser effectively cleanses the skin without stripping away the natural lipids. When treating photoaged skin, a mild cream-based cleanser is recommended.

2. **Growth factors**
   Fibroblast growth factor products stimulate fibroblast synthesis of collagen and other ECM components. They typically contain fibroblast-secreted substances such as epidermal growth factor, transforming growth factor beta and platelet-derived growth factor. Growth factor products may be obtained from a variety of sources, including fibroblasts in neonatal human foreskin or recombinant human epidermal growth factor engineered from yeast and bacteria. A growth factor product is often incorporated into a daily skin care regimen to improve skin hydration and reduce roughness, hyperpigmentation and wrinkles in photoaged skin.

3. **Retinoids**

   Topical retinoids are vitamin A derivatives and analogues, which range from potent prescription products, such as tretinoin and tretinoin derivatives such as tazarotene, to less active cosmeceutical products, such as retinol and retinaldehyde (see Topical Skin Care Products section, Fig. 1). Retinoids promote healthy epidermal turn over and proper skin function through reducing corneocyte cohesion and enhancing desquamation, inhibiting melanogenesis, antioxidant functions, stimulating collagen production, and reducing keratinization within hair follicles (i.e., clogged pores). They treat many aspects of photoaging including roughness, fine lines, sallowness, and hyperpigmentation. While prescription retinoids (e.g., tretinoin) are highly effective for rejuvenating skin, they are not easily combined with exfoliation treatments and other skin rejuvenation procedures. Therefore, prescription retinoids are often utilized as stand-alone skin care treatments and non-prescription retinoids, such as retinol, are preferred products which can be incorporated into the Topical Product Regimen for Photoaged Skin.

4. **Moisturizers**

   Moisturizer products hydrate the skin and in doing so can temporarily improve the skin's appearance by reducing wrinkles. Consistent use may achieve long-lasting effects by restoring barrier function. In addition, moisturizers also function as the vehicles for delivery of active ingredients to the skin, as all topical products are formulated in some kind of moisturizer base. Moisturizer formulations vary in their hydrating capabilities and range from very hydrating ointments and creams, to less hydrating lotions, serums, and gels. Selection of a moisturizer formulation is based on the hydration status of patients' skin which ranges from dry to oily. Photoaged skin is typically normal to dry and lotions or creams are preferred product formulations for daily regimens.

5. **Antioxidants**

   Topical antioxidants are used to reduce the harmful oxidative effects of UV radiation on skin. UV exposure initiates multiple changes within epidermal skin cells, including formation of highly reactive atoms and molecules, referred to as free radicals. There are many types of free radicals and reactive oxygen species (which include hydroxyl radicals, superoxide anions and nitric oxide) are the most widely studied in skin care because of the significant role they play in cutaneous damage. Topical use of an antioxidant product can assist in the prevention and reversal of cellular oxidation and, ultimately, the prevention and treatment of visible signs of aging. An antioxidant product such as a serum containing vitamin C and E is an essential component of the daily Topical Product Regimen for photoaged skin.

6. **Sunscreens**

   Sunscreens protect skin by reducing UV exposure. The most effective sunscreen products are broad-spectrum, offering protection from both UVA and UVB radiation, and maintain stability when exposed to sunlight. Sunscreen ingredients are classified as either chemical or physical (although technically all sunscreen ingredients are chemicals). Chemical sunscreens are organic substances that protect cells by absorbing UV radiation. Physical sunscreens are inorganic mineral compounds such as titanium dioxide and zinc oxide, that offer protection by reflecting, scattering, and to some degree, absorbing, UV radiation.

   Choosing a topical product line for incorporation into a practice can be challenging, as there are many options available. In addition, cosmetic products (including cosmeceuticals) are not regulated by the U.S. Food and Drug Administration (FDA) and, therefore, are not required to have evidence supporting their safety or efficacy.

Furthermore, the lack of peer-reviewed, blinded studies makes standard methods of medical product evaluation difficult. A basic knowledge of skin care ingredients, as evidence-based as possible, is essential to evaluating and selecting products for the office-setting.

One of the main decisions in selecting topical products for the office setting is whether to select a comprehensive single product line from one company, or to have products from many companies. Carrying a single skin care line has the advantage of product compatibility and logistic simplicity with ordering from one source. However, certain skin care companies may excel in only a small number of products which may not adequately meet patients' needs. Dispensing multiple skin care product lines from an office can be a more complex process, but, it may allow the provider flexibility in selecting a wide variety of products. In either case, it is important that the provider and staff are well versed in the products and their ingredients to create the most effective regimens and help ensure that particular ingredients are not overused.

Patient Selection

Exfoliation procedures and regular use of skin care products benefit almost any patient with regard to skin health and appearance, with few exceptions (see contraindications below). Patients exhibiting mild to moderate photoaging changes with rough skin texture, fine lines, and uneven pigmentation are ideal candidates. They typically demonstrate improvements after a series of exfoliation treatments and consistent topical product use over 3–6 months. Patients with moderate to severe photoaged skin may require combination treatments with laser or intense pulsed light (IPL) technologies to achieve significant improvements. Setting realistic expectations, and discussing achievable results during the consultation process is essential to success with office skin care treatments and patient satisfaction.

Aesthetic Consultation

During consultation the patient's medical history is reviewed, including: medications, allergies, past medical history such as herpes eruptions in the treatment area and conditions contraindicating treatment (see below), cosmetic history such as current skin care regimen, minimally invasive procedures, and plastic surgeries. Repeated dissatisfaction with prior aesthetic treatments can be a marker for patients with body dysmorphic disorder or unrealistic expectations, which are contraindications for aesthetic treatment. An example of an aesthetic intake form that may be used is shown in Appendix 2, Patient Intake Form.

A skin analysis is performed to determine the patient's Fitzpatrick skin type and Glogau score (see below). The skin is examined to assess for hydration (see below), the presence of lesions and problem areas such as hyperpigmentation, acne papules, pustules and comedones, erythema, telangiectasias, seborrheic keratoses, sebaceous hyperplasia, actinic keratoses, and lesions suspicious for skin cancers. Findings are typically documented in writing and photographically. An example of a Skin Analysis form that may be used is provided in Appendix 3.

Treatment options are discussed, including the number of recommended treatments, anticipated results with realistic expectations and costs. A cosmetic treatment plan is collaboratively formulated with the patient and recorded in the chart.

Fitzpatrick Skin Type

The Fitzpatrick scale is a means of assessing the skin's coloration and visible reaction to the sun. Skin types I–III are typically Caucasian, IV–V have olive or light brown skin tones such as people of Mediterranean, Asian and Latin descent, and VI are black, typically of African-American descent (Fig. 20). Fitzpatrick skin type determination may be used to guide the aggressiveness of aesthetic treatments and as a gross predictor of treatment response. For example, patients with lighter skin types (I–III) can typically tolerate more aggressive treatments and have low risks of pigmentary changes. Patients with darker skin types (IV–VI) have greater risks of undesired pigmentary changes, such as hyperpigmentation, and require more conservative treatments to reduce the likelihood of these complications.

Glogau Classification of Photoaging

The Glogau classification is used to assess the severity of photoaging, especially with regard to wrinkles (Fig. 21). This baseline measure is determined at the time of consultation and may be used to guide therapy. In general, Glogau types I–III tend

Fitzpatrick skin type	Skin color	Reaction to sun	
I	very white or freckled	always burns	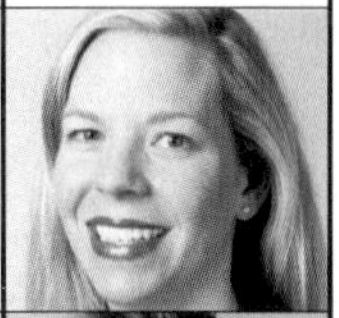
II	white	usually burns	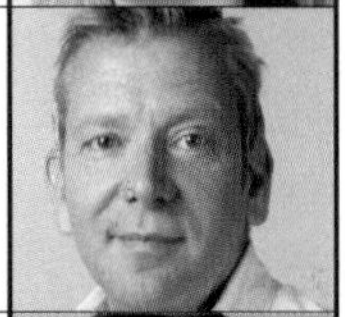
III	white to olive	sometimes burns	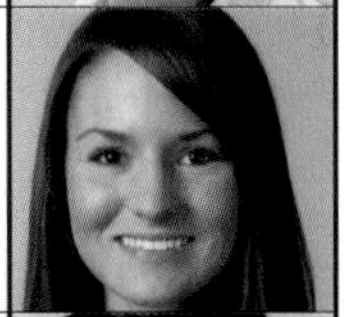
IV	brown	rarely burns	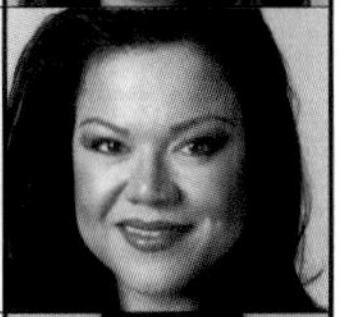
V	dark brown	very rarely burns	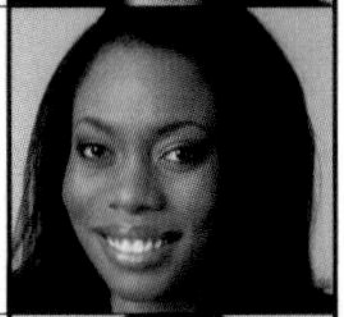
VI	black	never burns	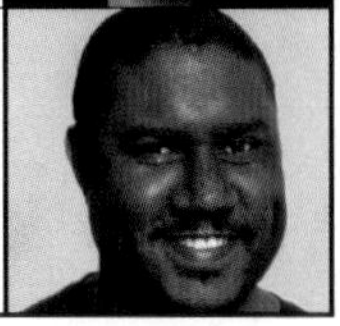

FIGURE 20 ● Fitzpatrick skin types. (Courtesy of PCA SKIN)

Type I Mild photoaging	Type II Moderate photoaging	Type III Advanced photoaging	Type IV Severe photoaging

• Mild pigmentary
  changes
 	
• No keratoses
 	
• Minimal or
  no wrinkles
	• Early solar lentigines
	
	• Rare keratoses,
	  mainly palpable
	
	• Wrinkles seen only
	  with facial expression
		• Obvious dyschromia
		  and telangiectasias
		
		• Visible keratoses
		
		• Wrinkles seen
		  at rest
			• Sallow (yellow-gray)
			  color
			
			• Keratoses and skin
			  malignancies
			
			• Wrinkles throughout,
			  little normal skin

Patient age: 20s	Patient age: 30s or 40s	Patient age: 50s	Patient age: 60s or 70s
Minimal or no makeup	Usually wears some foundation	Always wears heavy foundation	Can't wear makeup - 'cakes and cracks'

FIGURE 21 ● Glogau classification.

to show the most noticeable improvements with exfoliation procedures and skin care products. Glogau type IV patients often require more aggressive skin treatments such as ablative laser resurfacing, dermal filler and botulinum toxin injections to yield significant results.

Skin Hydration Levels

Skin hydration may be clinically described as normal, dry, or oily, and is often referred to by patients as their "skin type." Skin hydration status can be determined by history and examination. Patients with dehydrated dry skin often report a tight sensation after cleansing and on examination have a dull complexion, and may have skin flaking. Patients with oily skin typically report shininess throughout the day, particularly in the forehead, nose, and chin ("T-zone"). Determining patients' skin hydration helps guide product selection, particularly with cleansers and moisturizers, as most companies define their products for use by skin hydration. Patients with photoaged skin usually suffer from dehydration.

Photodocumentation

Photographs are recommended prior to treatment, midway through a series of treatments, and posttreatment. Consistent lighting and positioning is important when documenting skin care treatments, as improvements are subtle and can be challenging to capture photographically. Patients are typically positioned for photographs fully upright looking straight ahead. Photographs are taken of the full face from the front, 45 degrees and 90 degrees and zoomed in on areas with specific findings.

Informed Consent

It is advisable to address all aspects of the informed consent process prior to performing treatment. Patients are educated the about the nature of their condition or aesthetic issues, and details of the proposed treatments and alternative treatments are reviewed. The potential benefits are discussed, along with realistic expectations, and possible complications associated with procedure, and adequate opportunity is provided for all questions to be answered. The informed consent process is documented and a signed consent form placed in the chart. An example of a consent form for skin care procedures and product use is shown in Appendix 4, Consent for Skin Care Treatments.

Indications for Skin Care Treatments

- Photodamage
- Rough texture
- Fine lines and wrinkles
- Hyperpigmentation
- Enlarged pores
- Acne simplex (comedonal) and acne vulgaris (papulopustular)*
- Superficial acne scarring
- Dull, sallow skin color
- Keratosis pilaris
- Thickened scaling skin (e.g., ichthyosis)
- Dry skin (xerosis)
- Seborrheic keratosis scaling
- Enhanced penetration of products

Aftercare for Skin Care Treatments

- Skin may feel sensitive, tight, and dry and appear pink or red.
- Cool compresses may be applied to the treatment area for 15 minutes every 1–2 hours as needed for discomfort. An OTC pain reliever such as acetaminophen or ibuprofen may be taken as directed, but is rarely necessary.
- For chemical peels, the degree of postprocedure skin peeling varies and is dependent on the peel used and preprocedure condition of the patient's skin. Skin peeling ranges from mild flaking to sheets of peeling skin. Lack of peeling does not indicate that the treatment was ineffective or too weak. Patients are advised to avoid picking, abrading or scrubbing skin that is sensitive or peeling to reduce the risk of scarring and postinflammatory hyperpigmentation.
- Postprocedure skin care products are recommended for 1–2 weeks after treatment that soothe skin and do not contain potentially irritating ingredients (see Skin Care Products for Pre and Post Procedures, Topical Skin Care Products section).
- Patients may resume their regular Topical Product Regimen once the skin has fully returned to normal, approximately 1–2 weeks after treatment.
- Patients are advised to avoid direct sun exposure for at least 4 weeks posttreatment to minimize complications.
- A broad-spectrum sunscreen, with an SPF of 30 or greater containing zinc oxide or titanium dioxide, is used daily.
- An example of a postprocedure patient handout is provided in Appendix 5, Before and After Instructions for Skin Care Treatments.

*Pustules are avoided with MDA.

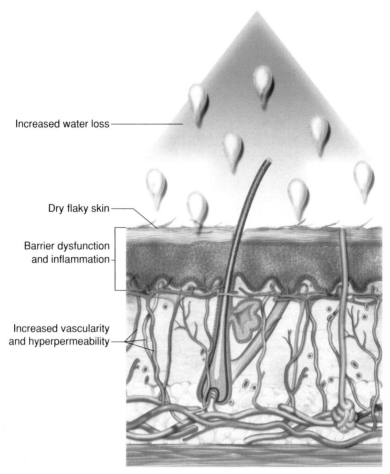

Increased water loss

Dry flaky skin

Barrier dysfunction and inflammation

Increased vascularity and hyperpermeability

FIGURE 22 ● Erythematous, sensitive skin pathophysiology.

Other Skin Conditions that can Benefit from Skin Care

Facial Erythema: Rosacea and Sensitive Skin

Facial erythema can be seen with a variety of dermatologic conditions including rosacea, sensitive skin, and photoaged skin. Erythema is typically evident in the medial face as telangiectasias, fine caliber vessels and/or background erythema. Almost all erythematous skin conditions have common underlying pathology with a dysfunctional skin barrier resulting in increased TEWL; as well as inflammation and associated increased vascularity with hyperpermeable and dilated capillaries (Fig. 22).

  Rosacea is a chronic sensitive skin condition that affects millions of Americans every year. It is seen most commonly in women between the ages of 30 and 50, yet men who are affected typically have more severe presentations. There are four subtypes of rosacea:

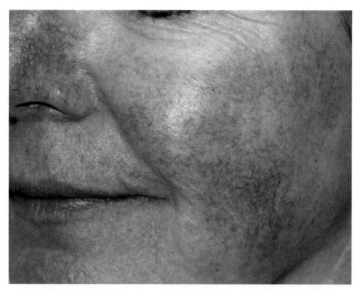

FIGURE 23 ● Rosacea type I (erythematotelangiectatic rosacea). (Courtesy of Rebecca Small, MD)

- Subtype 1 (erythematotelangiectatic) presents as background erythema and telangiectasias on the convexities of the face (forehead, cheeks, nose, and chin) (Fig. 23).
- Subtype 2 (papulopustular) presents with papule- and pustule-like lesions within the borders of the erythematous areas as defined above (Fig. 24).
- Subtype 3 (phymatous) is marked by a thickening of the skin, most commonly affecting the nose (rhinophyma). This subtype typically affects men more than women.
- Subtype 4 (ocular) affects the eyes and eyelids, and usually presents with conjunctival hyperemia and blepharitis.

Frequent and prolonged flushing, the hallmark signs of rosacea, can be triggered by many different factors such as weather extremes, consumption of alcoholic or hot beverages, emotional stress, spicy foods, and irritating topical products. Many theories have been proposed for the etiology of rosacea, but as yet there is no single definitive cause. Some common theories include upregulation of cytokines that lead to flushing, chronic inflammation and vascular dilation, and proliferation of the demodex mite with excessive inflammatory response to colonization.

Therapies for facial erythema are aimed at supporting and stabilizing the skin barrier, replenishing moisture and reducing inflammation. Nonirritating topical products are recommended that have low concentrations of active ingredients (see Topical Product Regimen for Facial Erythema: Rosacea and Sensitive Skin section, in Topical Skin Care Products).

The use of exfoliation procedures such as chemical peels and MDA with erythematous skin is controversial. These treatments have the potential to irritate and inflame skin; however, the epidermal barrier may ultimately be improved resulting in overall, clinical improvement. References and management strategies for rosacea in this book are primarily for subtypes I and II.

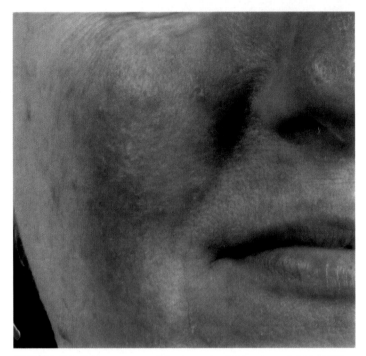

FIGURE 24 ● Rosacea type II (acne rosacea). (Courtesy of PCA SKIN)

Acne

Acne is one of the most common dermatologic disorders, affecting nearly 50 million patients in the United States. It is a chronic skin condition and presents with many different types of lesions, described below.

Acne Lesions

- **Open comedones** are commonly referred to as 'blackheads' by patients (Fig. 25). They represent the presence of keratin and sebum within a hair follicle. They can be extracted by applying gentle pressure around the follicle; however, they almost always reoccur.
- **Closed comedones** are small flesh-colored lesions commonly referred to as 'whiteheads'. They are caused by a buildup of keratin and sebum that is trapped within the follicle by overlying skin cells (Fig. 26). Closed comedones respond best to exfoliation, rather than extraction. Open and closed comedones are most common in oilier areas of the face, including the nose, forehead and chin.
- **Papules** are small, solid, inflamed bumps that are red in color and do not contain pus (Fig. 27). Papules should not be extracted. They often progress in to pustules, which can then be extracted.
- **Pustules** are small inflamed bumps that are red in color and contain pus, which is visible as a white tip (Fig. 27). Pustules can be extracted by applying light pressure to the base of the lesions. If necessary, a lancet may be used to create a small puncture in the lesion to ease extraction.

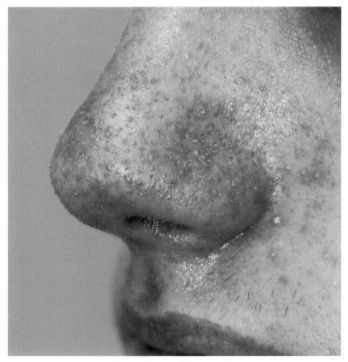

FIGURE 25 ● Acne simplex with open comedones, closed comedones and a pustule. (Courtesy of Rebecca Small, MD)

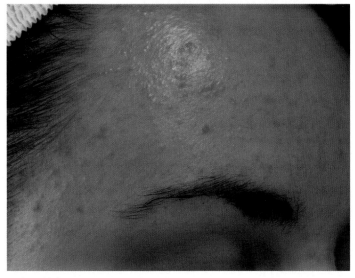

FIGURE 26 ● Acne simplex with closed comedones. (Courtesy of PCA SKIN)

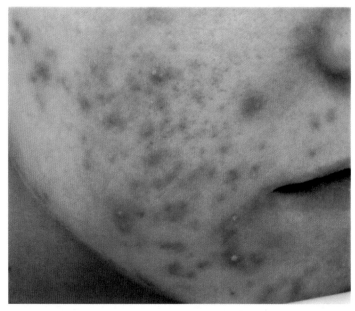

FIGURE 27 ● Acne vulgaris with extensive inflamed papules and pustules. (Courtesy of PCA SKIN)

- **Nodules and cysts** are collections beneath the surface of the skin that occur when sebaceous glands become inflamed and infected (Fig. 28). They usually cause discomfort. Extraction is not recommended because of the depth of the lesion. They may result in scarring or cellulitis, especially if extraction or picking is attempted.

Acne Classification

Acne classification is based on the presence of inflammatory lesions. Acne simplex has minimal to no inflammatory lesions, and acne vulgaris has inflammatory lesions.

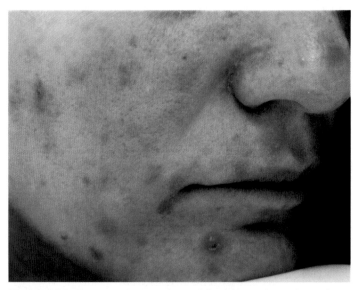

FIGURE 28 ● Acne vulgaris with rare inflamed papules and pustules and chin cyst. (Courtesy of PCA SKIN)

Acne can be further classified by grade based on the predominant lesion type, as described below.

Acne Simplex—Non-inflammatory

- Grade I—Comedonal lesions
- Grade II—Comedonal lesions and with occasional papular and pustular lesions that are rarely inflamed

Acne Vulgaris—Inflammatory

- Grade III—Comedonal, papular, and pustular lesions with significant inflammation and bacteria present
- Grade IV—Comedonal, papular, pustular, nodular, and cystic lesions with significant bacteria present

The pathophysiologic factors contributing to acne formation, regardless of the grade include: (1) abnormal exfoliation and hyperkeratinization within hair follicles leading to clogged pores, open comedones, and closed comedones, (2) increased sebum production, (3) overgrowth of Propionibacterium acnes (P. acnes) bacteria in obstructed pores leading to (4) inflammatory papules, pustules, nodules, and cysts.

Other Factors Contributing to Acne Formation

- **Hormonal fluctuations** can increase sebum production. Follicles contain androgen receptors and elevated relative testosterone levels can increase the size of sebaceous glands and the amount of sebum secreted. Acne is most common in male patients during puberty when testosterone levels peak. Female patients can experience acne breakouts related to the menstrual cycle, which usually occur immediately preceding and during menstruation. At this time in the cycle, testosterone levels are high relative to progesterone and estrogen that are diminished.
- **Stress** triggers the release of cortisol which stimulates sebum production and inflammation. Acne patients have demonstrably higher cortisol levels and although stress is not a direct cause of acne, it is thought to worsen the condition.
- **Comedogenic topical products** clog pores and can trigger acne. Comedogenicity relates to the propensity to cause acne, and is determined by the formulation of a finished product rather than single ingredients. Many products are labeled as "noncomedogenic"; however, this is not an FDA recognized term nor is there any standardization in testing. "Noncomedogenic" products can, therefore, be comedogenic.
- **Over-drying** the skin can trigger acne. While the goal of acne treatment is to control sebum production, stripping the skin of all hydration can actually stimulate sebum production and inflammation, thereby increasing acne.

Treatment of acne is guided by the type of lesions present and the overall severity of the condition. All topical regimens for the treatment of acne utilize exfoliants and products which decrease sebum production. Therapies for inflammatory acne also include antibacterials against P. acnes and products with anti-inflammatory properties (see the Topical Product Regimen for Acne, Topical Skin Care Products section). Superficial exfoliation with chemical peels and/or MDA are also utilized, as exfoliation assists in keeping the follicle clear of debris and bacteria, and allows for better penetration of topical products. In addition, exfoliation procedures can also reduce postinflammatory hyperpigmentation, improving the overall appearance of patient's skin and self-confidence.

Acne in Ethnic Skin

Acne is one of the most common skin conditions affecting patients of Latino, African-American, and Asian backgrounds, and sequelae are often more severe in darker skin types (i.e., Fitzpatrick Skin Types IV–VI). While the pathology of acne does not vary by ethnicity, lesion characteristics may differ. Comedonal acne in African-American skin tends to exhibit significantly higher amounts of inflammation than comedonal acne in Caucasian skin. Asian and Indian skin have a greater propensity towards papular lesions. Ethnic skin is more prone to pigmentary changes such as postinflammatory hyperpigmentation (PIH). Therefore, it is important to treat the skin without over-stimulation; which means using less irritating products and more anti-inflammatory ingredients. It is common for patients to think that their PIH is scarring, which is not the case. If PIH is present, ingredients capable of inhibiting melanogenesis, such as hydroquinone, can also be incorporated into their regimen.

Hyperpigmentation

Hyperpigmentation is due to increased melanin synthesis and deposition in the skin. There are many skin conditions that present with hyperpigmentation, and hyperpigmentation associated with photoaging is one of the most common. Chronic UV exposure contributes to formation of lentigines, mottled pigmentation, and darkened freckles (also called ephelides). Chronic UV exposure can also result in Poikiloderma of Civatte, which is mottled pigmentation associated with erythema, typically seen on the sides of the neck, cheeks, and chest. Other common cosmetic hyperpigmentation conditions include melasma and postinflammatory hyperpigmentation.

The underlying pathophysiologic mechanism for disorders of hyperpigmentation is overproduction of melanin. The key regulatory step in melanin synthesis (melanogenesis) occurs in melanocytes and is the conversion of tyrosine to melanin by the enzyme tyrosinase. Melanocyte stimulating hormone (MSH) initiates this enzymatic conversion. Melanin is packaged into melanosomes within the melanocytes, transported along the melanocytes dendrites, and then distributed to surrounding epidermal keratinocytes. A lentigo, for example, is a collection of melanin filled keratinocytes and corneocytes that are formed by UV-stimulated melanocytes (Fig. 29). Many factors, in addition to UV exposure, can upregulate melanin synthesis contributing to unwanted hyperpigmentation (Fig. 17).

Melasma, also referred to as chloasma, is characterized by hyperpigmented patches and macules. Centrofacial distribution on the forehead, cheeks, upper lip, and nose is common (Fig. 30) and mandibular involvement may also be seen. Melasma is frequently observed following a change in female hormonal status such as during pregnancy (chloasma) or with use of oral contraceptives. As with all hyperpigmentation disorders, melasma is exacerbated by UV exposure.

Postinflammatory hyperpigmentation is visible as brown macules at sites of previously inflamed acne lesions or sites of wound healing (Fig. 31). Patients with darker Fitzpatrick skin types (IV–VI) are more susceptible to PIH, as are patients (of any skin type) with prolonged postprocedure erythma.

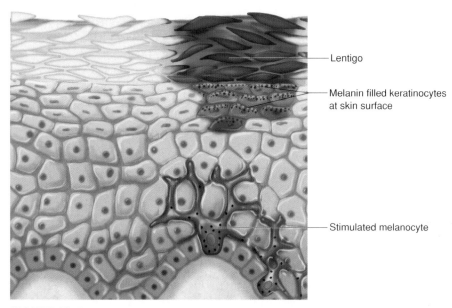

FIGURE 29 ● Hyperpigmented skin pathophysiology.

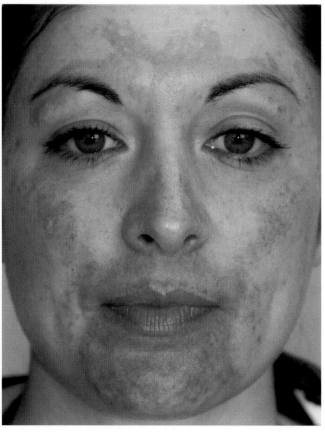

FIGURE 30 ● Melasma. (Courtesy of Rebecca Small, MD)

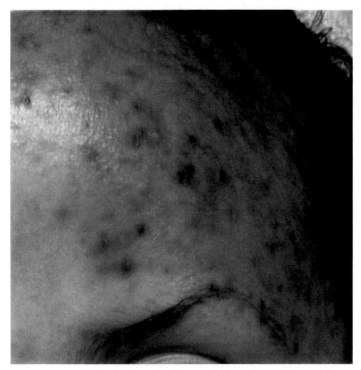

FIGURE 31 ● Postinflammatory hyperpigmentation. (Courtesy of PCA SKIN)

Treatment of hyperpigmentation includes superficial exfoliation with chemical peels and MDA to increase epidermal turnover and remove melanin-laden corneocytes. Topical products include sunscreen to reduce UV exposure, and melanogenesis inhibitors such as tyrosinase inhibitors (see Topical Product Regimen for Hyperpigmentation, Topical Skin Care Products section).

Combining Aesthetic Procedures

This practical guide provides an integrated approach for the treatment of sun-damaged skin utilizing a combination of superficial chemical peels, microdermabrasion, and a daily home skin care regimen. For patients with moderate to severe photoaged skin or those who desire enhanced results, MDA and chemical peels may be combined with other minimally invasive aesthetic procedures such as lasers, IPL, botulinum toxin, and/or dermal filler treatments.

Combining Microdermabrasion with Laser Photorejuvenation Treatments

Photorejuvenation is the treatment of hyperpigmentation and facial erythema in photoaged skin using non-ablative lasers or IPL devices. These treatments are based on the principle of selective photothermolysis. Chromophores, or light absorbing pigments in the skin, selectively absorb laser light energy, which is converted to heat in the targeted lesions. The lesions are heated, damaged and eliminated, while the surrounding skin is left unaffected. The two chromophores targeted in the skin during photorejuvenation treatments are melanin in pigmented lesions, and oxyhemoglobin in red vascular lesions.

When treating **hyperpigmentation**, such as lentigines, the melanin chromophore within the melanosomes of epidermal melanocytes and keratinocytes are targeted by the light energy, which then heats and ruptures the melanosomes. The treated lentigines typically darken for several days after treatment and form microcrusts which gradually flake off, exposing lightened or resolved lesions resulting in an even skin tone. MDA is often performed 2 weeks afterward to enhance results by accelerating exfoliation and removing any remaining darkened pigmentation from the photorejuvenation treatment.

When treating **facial erythema**, such as telangiectasias, the chromophore oxyhemoglobin within the blood vessel is targeted by light energy, which then heats and coagulates blood and closes the vessel lumen. The treated vascularities typically resolve within a few days. MDA can be performed immediately prior to photorejuvenation treatment to enhance results. The intent is to temporarily increase blood flow and the intensity of erythema so that the laser or IPL device has more target and greater treatment efficacy.

Combining Microdermabrasion and Chemical Peels with Non-ablative Collagen Stimulating Lasers

This approach to skin rejuvenation targets both the dermis and epidermis to enhance results for treatment of fine lines and enlarged pores. Collagen synthesis in the dermis is stimulated with a non-ablative laser (e.g., Q-switch 1064 nm laser) or IPL. Exfoliation of the epidermis can be performed consecutively in the same visit using MDA as well as a chemical peel. This combination treatment can be performed monthly for cumulative results.

Combining Skin Care Treatments and Products with Dermal Filler and Botulinum Toxin Procedures

Patients with moderate to severe sun-damaged skin often exhibit deeper static lines and wrinkles which MDA, chemical peels, and skin care products may not effectively address. Utilizing dermal fillers can restore the volume loss, reduce static lines, and redefine facial contours. If dynamic lines are present, due to hyperdynamic muscle contraction, botulinum toxin treatments are recommended. MDA may be performed immediately prior to botulinum toxin or dermal filler treatments in the same visit. Superficial chemical peels may also be performed immediately prior to botulinum toxin treatments; however, it is advisable to wait until all skin flaking is resolved before performing dermal filler treatments.

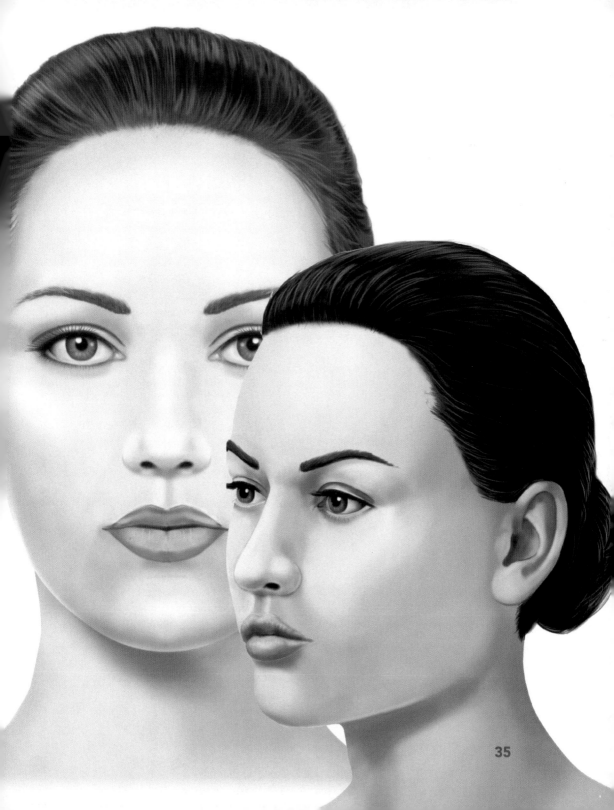

Chemical Peels

Chapter 1

Chemical Peel Introduction and Foundation Concepts

Chemical peel treatments, also referred to as chemexfoliation, remove the outer layers of skin to improve overall skin function and enhance appearance. Their mechanism of action is based on the principles of wound healing whereby, controlled wounding of the skin with removal of skin layers helps to stimulate cell renewal, and regenerate a healthier epidermis and dermis. This Practical Guide focuses primarily on the use of superficial* chemical peels to treat photodamaged skin and other common dermatologic conditions such as sensitive skin, acne and hyperpigmentation. Superficial peels have few risks of complications and can be readily combined with microdermabrasion treatments, topical home care products and other aesthetic procedures to maximize outcomes and tailor treatments to patients' specific needs and conditions.

Patient Selection

Patients with mild to moderate photoaging changes such as solar lentigines, dullness and rough skin texture (e.g., Glogau types I and II), and acneic conditions, typically derive the most noticeable benefits with superficial chemical peels (see Introduction Concepts and Foundation Concepts for a description of Glogau types). Fine lines, enlarged pores, and atrophic scars can also be improved with superficial peels; however, results are not comparable to those achieved with deeper skin resurfacing procedures, such as medium depth peels or laser resurfacing. Assessment of patients' expectations at the time of consultation and commitment to a series of peels is essential to ensure success with superficial chemical peels.

Superficial peels can be used in all skin types (Fitzpatrick I–VI) (see Introduction Concepts and Foundation Concepts for a description of Fitzpatrick skin types). However, patients with darker skin types (IV–VI) have greater risks of postinflammatory hyperpigmentation (PIH). Patients with severe cases of erythematous conditions including rosacea, telangiectasias and Poikiloderma of Civatte have a risk of erythema exacerbation. While superficial peels can be used in these groups, less aggressive treatments are advised to the reduce risks of PIH and erythema exacerbation respectively.

References to superficial chemical peels also include very superficial chemical peels, unless otherwise indicated.

Indications

- Photodamage
- Rough texture
- Fine lines
- Hyperpigmentation
- Dull, sallow skin color
- Enlarged pores
- Acne simplex (comedonal) and acne vulgaris (papulopustular)
- Acne scars
- Keratosis pilaris
- Thickened scaling skin (e.g., icthyosis)
- Dry skin (xerosis)
- Seborrheic keratosis scaling
- Enhanced penetration of topical products

While the superficial peels discussed in this chapter are appropriate for the indications listed above, some subtle trends for selecting one peel over another exist with regard to indication (see Chemical Peel Selection below).

Chemical Peel Classification

Chemical peels can be classified based on their depth of penetration into the skin as follows: very superficial, superficial, medium and deep (see Anatomy, Fig. 4).

- **Very superficial** peels penetrate the **stratum corneum** and possibly the upper layers of the stratum spinosum in the epidermis
- **Superficial** peels penetrate the **entire epidermis** and possibly the papillary dermis
- **Medium** depth peels penetrate through the entire epidermis and possibly the **upper reticular dermis**
- **Deep** peels penetrate the **midreticular dermis**

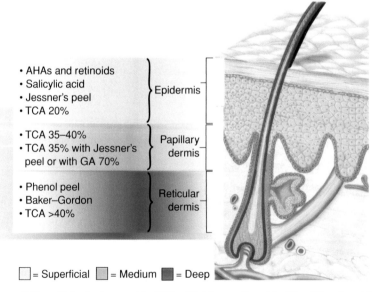

• AHAs and retinoids
• Salicylic acid
• Jessner's peel
• TCA 20%
} Epidermis

• TCA 35–40%
• TCA 35% with Jessner's peel or with GA 70%
} Papillary dermis

• Phenol peel
• Baker–Gordon
• TCA >40%
} Reticular dermis

☐ = Superficial ▨ = Medium ▪ = Deep

AHAs = Alpha hydroxy acids TCA = Trichloroacetic acid GA = Glycolic acid

FIGURE 1 ● Depth of skin resurfacing with superficial, medium, and deep chemical peels.

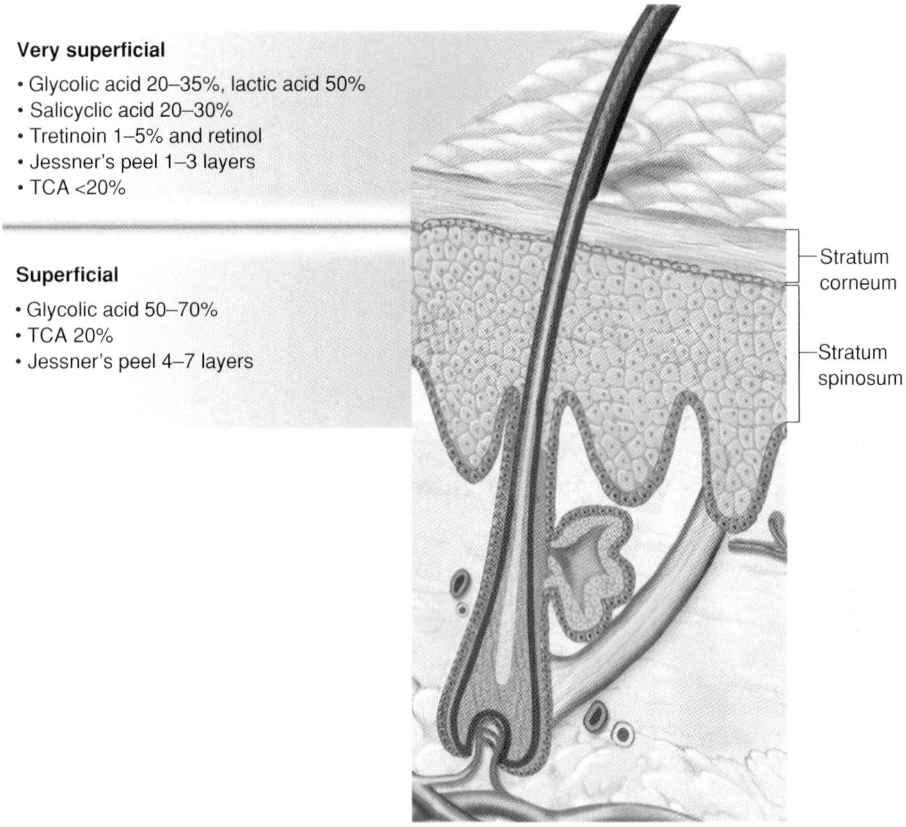

Very superficial

- Glycolic acid 20–35%, lactic acid 50%
- Salicyclic acid 20–30%
- Tretinoin 1–5% and retinol
- Jessner's peel 1–3 layers
- TCA <20%

Superficial

- Glycolic acid 50–70%
- TCA 20%
- Jessner's peel 4–7 layers

Stratum corneum

Stratum spinosum

TCA = Trichloroacetic acid

FIGURE 2 ● Depth of skin resurfacing with very superficial and superficial chemical peels.

Common superficial chemical peels and their typical depth of skin penetration (also referred to as resurfacing depth) are shown in Figures 1 and 2. Many factors influence a chemical peel's depth of penetration, and although a given chemical peel may be classified as a superficial peeling agent, in practice, the depth of penetration may vary. Figures 1 and 2, therefore, serve only as general guides for chemical peel depths.

Factors Influencing the Depth of Chemical Peel Penetration

The type of chemical agent used is the main determinant of resurfacing depth. Many other factors also affect the depth of resurfacing and are listed below.

- Chemical peel agent
- Concentration
- Acid pH
- Application time (i.e., the amount of time a peel is left on the skin prior to neutralization—for those peels requiring neutralization)
- Application technique (e.g., pressure applied to the skin and type of applicator)
- Quantity applied (e.g., the number of layers, where a layer is defined as continuous coverage of the treatment area)
- Skin preparation (e.g., previous skin resurfacing procedures and topical products used prior to the procedure)
- Skin characteristics (e.g., thick sebaceous or thin dry skin)

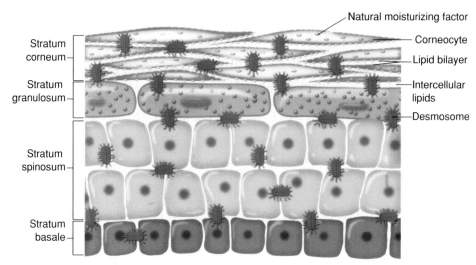

Stratum corneum — Natural moisturizing factor / Corneocyte / Lipid bilayer
Stratum granulosum — Intercellular lipids / Desmosome
Stratum spinosum
Stratum basale

FIGURE 3 ● Skin desmosomal intercellular bonds.

The depth of penetration for a given chemical peel agent is increased by a higher concentration, lower pH, longer application time, greater pressure, more layers of product, preprocedure use of topical products (such as retinoids and hydroxy acids) or recent exfoliation (such as microdermabrasion) which thin or remove the stratum corneum barrier, and non-intact skin (such as acne papules).

Mechanism of Action

Chemical peels remove the outer skin layers through keratolysis and keratocoagulation. Keratolytic agents, such as lactic and glycolic acids, penetrate through the stratum corneum and disrupt corneocyte adhesion by breaking intercellular desmosomal bonds (Fig. 3). Keratocoagulants, such as TCA, destroy surface cells through protein denaturation and keratinocyte coagulation. The effect on the skin with either mechanism is desquamation and acceleration of the epidermal renewal process.

Neutralization

Some chemical peel acids require termination of activity through neutralization. Neutralization is performed by applying a base such as sodium bicarbonate solution (10–15%), to the skin, or by applying water to dilute the acid, which raises the pH and renders the acid ineffective. For example, glycolic acid remains active in the epidermis if neutralization is not performed and can continue to penetrate into the skin. Once a base is applied, glycolic acid is neutralized and its effects terminated.

Other acids, referred to as 'self-neutralizing acids', do not require application of a base for termination of activity. The activity of self-neutralizing acids is spontaneously terminated shortly after application by the water and other components in the skin, which effectively dilute and neutralize the acid. TCA is an example of a self-neutralizing acid.

The requirement for neutralization is usually inherent in the type of acid. However, product formulation and acid concentration can also affect the need for neutralization. For example, glycolic acid always requires neutralization and TCA is always self-neutralizing, regardless of their concentrations. Lactic acid, however, varies in its requirement for neutralization. In low concentrations such as 15%, lactic acid is self-neutralizing. In higher concentrations such as 45%, lactic acid requires neutralization by application of a base. Following manufacturer protocols for specific products is important for using chemical peels safely and effectively.

Basic Versus Advanced Chemical Peels

This text focuses on basic chemical peel agents used for superficial peeling, which primarily involve wounding of the epidermis. These peels may be performed with regularity to promote healthy skin and enhance appearance, have few risks of complications, and can be readily combined with other aesthetic procedures. Medium and deep peels that penetrate into the dermis are considered advanced chemical peels. They offer greater skin rejuvenation benefits; however, medium and deep peels also have greater risks of adverse outcomes and long-term complications. In addition, advanced peels are appropriate for a limited patient population, require more intense postprocedure care, and some may only be performed once or twice in a lifetime.

Chemical Peel Products

Alpha Hydroxy Acids

Alpha hydroxy acids (AHAs) are some of the first agents that were used for chemical peeling. They are primarily derived from fruits and include glycolic (sugarcane), malic (apples), tartaric (grapes), citric (citrus), mandelic (almonds), lactic (milk), and phytic (rice) acids. AHAs penetrate into the stratum corneum and cause desquamation by breaking corneocyte desmosomal bonds. AHAs are also used in topical products as part of daily skin care regimens in low concentrations (10% or less) and in less acidic preparations (pH 3.5 or greater).

Glycolic acid (GA) is the most commonly used AHA. Glycolic acid peels are typically clear colorless solutions or gels that do not change in appearance upon application to the skin. As there is not a reliable visible clinical endpoint with GA peels, application must be timed and the acid neutralized at the appropriate point to control the procedure. Clinical response to glycolic acid can be variable. For example, some patients have an intense inflammatory response to low strength (20–35%) short duration applications (1–3 minutes), while others tolerate high strengths (70%) for longer duration (up to 7 minutes). Minimal to no skin flaking or peeling is evident postprocedure with GA peels.

GA is found in concentrations up to 70% in superficial chemical peels which typically have a pH of 2.5 to 3. Formulations with lower pHs and higher concentrations have stronger biologic effects. However, very low pHs (pH < 2) can be associated with greater risks of vesiculation, necrosis and crusting and do not offer improved results over less acidic preparations.

Lactic acid (LA) is one of the more gentle acids and is inherently hydrating. After application to the skin, lactic acid forms lactate which is a component of the skin's natural moisturizing factor that functions as a humectant. Lactic acid is used as a very superficial peeling agent in concentrations up to 50% and is frequently combined with other superficial peeling agents in blended peels.

Beta Hydroxy Acids

Salicylic acid (SA) is derived from willow tree bark, wintergreen oil and sweet birch. SA is a beta hydroxy acid and is found in concentrations up to 30% in superficial peels. Its lipophilic properties enable SA to penetrate and dissolve sebum, making it a

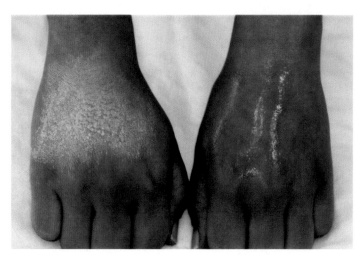

FIGURE 4 ● Salicylic acid (on the left) produces a white precipitate or pseudofrost and glycolic acid (on the right) is clear and colorless. (Courtesy of Rebecca Small, MD)

highly effective therapy for acne. In addition, it has anti-inflammatory effects which make it suitable for sensitive skin conditions, such as rosacea. **β-lipohydroxy acid (LHA)** is a newer peel, derived from SA, which has greater lipophilicity compared to SA.

Salicylic acid has a mild anesthetic effect and compared to AHAs, SA peels produce less stinging upon application. Many SA peel products have a visible clinical endpoint on the skin with a fine white powder ('pseudofrost') which is a salt precipitate of salicylic acid. Figure 4 shows salicylic acid on the dorsum of one hand with its characteristic white precipitate and glycolic acid on the other hand. Salicylic acid peels are self-neutralizing and once the white powdery precipitate has formed, there is no further penetration of the acid into the skin. Salicylic acid is available as pure or combination peels and clinical endpoints vary based on the product used. For example, Jessner's peel (salicylic acid 14%, resorcinol 14% and lactic acid 14%) forms a white precipitate; whereas SkinCeutical's Salicylic/Mandelic Peel (salicylic acid 20% and mandelic acid 10%) does not form a white precipitate.

Trichloroacetic Acid

Trichloroacetic acid (TCA) is synthetically produced from acetic acid and chlorine. The resurfacing depth achieved with TCA ranges from superficial to deep depending on the acid concentration. It is commonly used as pure TCA in concentrations up to 20% for superficial peels. The Obagi Blue Peel, which derives its name from dye in the formulation that causes a temporary blue skin discoloration, contains TCA 20%, glycerin and saponins which slow penetration and release of TCA in the skin. TCA is also commonly used in blended superficial peels such as TCA 20% with LA 10%, and TCA 15% with SA 15%.

When applied topically, TCA causes visible whitening of the skin, referred to as frosting. Histologically, frosting corresponds to coagulation of epidermal proteins and keratinocytes. The degree of frosting directly corresponds to the TCA depth of penetration in the skin. Level I frosting is the desired clinical endpoint for superficial peeling, and is visible as faint skin whitening with patchy erythema. Figure 5 demonstrates

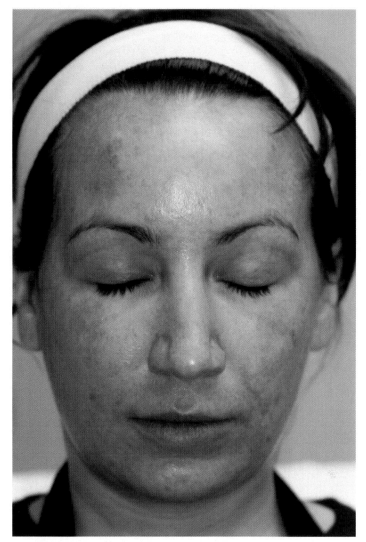

FIGURE 5 ● TCA 20% chemical peel immediately after application of 2 layers showing level I frosting. (Courtesy of Rebecca Small, MD)

level I frosting after 2 layers of TCA 20%. Level II frosting, visible as skin whitening with some erythema, corresponds to medium depth peeling. Level III frosting, visible as opaque whitening, corresponds to deep peeling. Unlike the white powdery pseudofrost of SA, true frosting cannot be wiped off the skin.

Higher strength pure TCA peels have more discomfort associated with application and more pronounced posttreatment desquamation compared to other superficial peels. Blended TCA peels, which have lower concentrations of TCA, are similar to other superficial peels with regard to discomfort and desquamation.

Jessner's and Other Blended Peels

Blended peels combine multiple acids in a single formulation. Most superficial peel agents are available in blended peel formulations, such as lactic acid/TCA, and salicylic acid/glycolic acid. By combining multiple acids, each can be used at a lower percentage, thereby maximizing outcomes and minimizing potential side effects from any one ingredient. Some blended peels also contain additional ingredients that target specific skin conditions such as melanogenesis inhibitors (e.g., hydroquinone and kojic acid), hydrating agents (e.g., soy isoflavones), anti-inflammatory (e.g., bisabolol) and antioxidant ingredients (e.g., L-ascorbic acid). A self-neutralizing peel containing TCA, lactic acid with melanogenesis inhibitors (Ultra Peel I by PCA SKIN) is an example of this type of enhanced blended peel.

Blended peels can be broken into two categories: requiring neutralization and self-neutralizing.

- **Blended peels requiring neutralization.** These peels require application of a base to terminate their activity. These peels typically contain glycolic acid or higher strength AHAs such as lactic acid 45%. Procedural instructions for blended peels requiring neutralization are similar to those for single ingredient glycolic acid peels and are reviewed in the Alpha Hydroxy Acid Peels: Glycolic Acid chapter.
- **Blended self-neutralizing peels.** Blended self-neutralizing peel effects are spontaneously terminated shortly after application to the skin. These peels often contain ingredients in the lower concentrations such as lactic acid 15% which are effectively diluted and neutralized by water and other components of the skin. Procedural instructions for self-neutralizing blended peels are reviewed in the Jessner's Peel chapter and Other Self-Neutralizing Blended Peels: Trichloroactetic Acid and Lactic Acid chapter.

Jessner's peel is a classic example of a blended self-neutralizing peel, which consists of lactic acid 14%, salicylic acid 14%, and resorcinol 14% in an alcohol base. Resorcinol is a phenol derivative and when used alone in high concentrations (greater than 50%) can be associated with toxicity such as myxedema and methemoglobinemia. Modified Jessner's peels are available that omit resorcinol. Enhanced Jessner's peels are also available that contain additional ingredients such as hydroquinone or kojic acid. After a Jessner's peel is applied, erythema is followed by a powdery whitening of the skin due to salicylic acid precipitate. Neutralization is not required and the white precipitate may be brushed off. Jessner's peels are frequently applied in multiple layers to increase the depth of penetration. Figure 6 shows a patient with mild erythema and a faint whitish coloration due to SA precipitate after 6 layers of a Jessner's peel.

Retinoids

Topical retinoids such as tretinoin (Retin-A) have long been components of home skin care regimens for the treatment of acne and skin rejuvenation. More recently, retinoids have been used as superficial peeling agents, ranging from prescription strength products such as retinoic acid (e.g., 0.3%) to lower strength products such as retinol (e.g., retinol 15%). Retinoic acid is the bioavailable form of vitamin A. It occurs naturally in rosehip seed oil, and is usually produced synthetically for topical use. Retinol, which is also synthetically produced, is converted to retinoic acid in the skin after application. All retinoids increase exfoliation by reducing corneocyte cohesion and stimulating epidermal cellular turnover. They also inhibit melanogenesis, increase collagen production, and reduce keratinization within hair follicles, making them beneficial for many skin conditions.

Retinoid peels can be used alone, but more often are used as 'booster' peels which are layered over other superficial peels, such as SA and GA, to intensify peel treatments and enhance desquamation. Retinoid peels leave a temporary yellow discoloration on the skin after application. Figure 7 shows a patient immediately after 6 layers of a Jessner's peel followed by 1 layer of a retinol 15% with lactic acid 15% peel showing

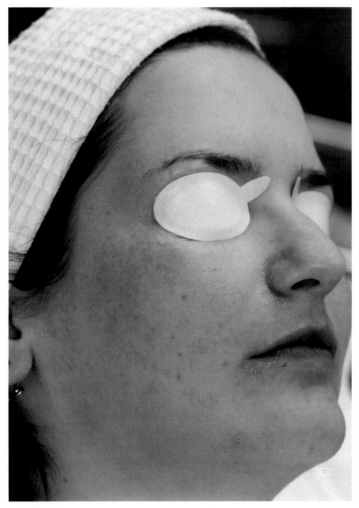

FIGURE 6 ● Jessner's peel immediately after application of 6 layers showing mild erythema and faint white skin coloration from the salicylic acid precipitate. (Courtesy of Rebecca Small, MD)

characteristic yellow skin discoloration. Retinoid peels do not require neutralization and are rinsed off by the patient 4–8 hours after application.

Enzymes

While most chemical peels are acids, proteolytic enzymes also exfoliate skin and are used for superficial chemical peeling. Most enzymes induce desquamation through keratolysis. Commonly used enzymes include bromelain (derived from pineapple), lactose (from sour milk), papain (from papaya), pepsin, pumpkin, tomato, and mushroom extracts. Due to their sources, enzyme products often have pungent odors.

Enzyme products are available in many different formulations (see below). Once applied to the skin, enzymes usually require activation by water. This may be accomplished by rubbing with moistened fingertips or using hot water in the form of steam or a warm moist towel after the product is applied to the skin. Patients typically experience a pleasant warming sensation, as opposed to the burning or stinging sensation associated with acids. Enzymes are usually applied for 2–10 minutes and then removed with water.

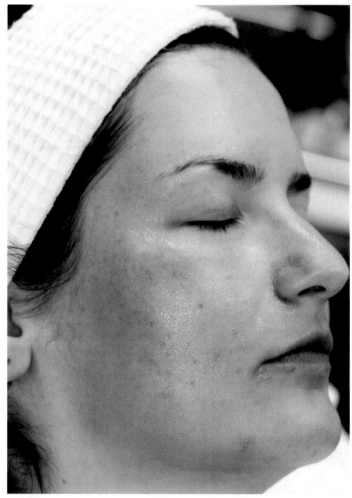

FIGURE 7 ● Retinoid peel (retinol 15% with lactic acid 15%) on top of a Jessner's peel (6 layers) immediately after application showing yellow skin coloration. (Courtesy of Rebecca Small, MD)

Chemical Peel Formulations

Chemical peel acids are available in many formulations including solutions, gels, and creams. Enzymes are formulated as powders, creams and gommages (Fig. 8). A gommage is a cream or paste that contains slightly sticky ingredients such as xanthan gum. After application to the skin it is allowed to dry, and then removed by rubbing which exfoliates the outermost layers of skin. Solutions have the advantage of requiring small amounts of product to cover the treatment area. Gels and creams offer more control due to their thicker consistency as they are less likely to drip or pool. Enzymes can require extended treatment times, particularly with powders that require reconstitution with water.

Chemical Peel Selection

All of the superficial peels discussed in this book may be used for rejuvenation of photodamaged skin. There are some subtle trends for selecting one peel over another

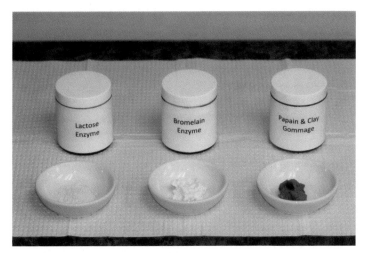

FIGURE 8 ● Enzymes product formulations: powder, cream, and gommage. (Courtesy of Rebecca Small, MD)

based on the properties of individual agents. Salicylic and glycolic acids and retinoids are often used for oily skin and acneic conditions; lactic acid for dehydration; mandelic, lactic and salicylic acid for sensitive skin and rosacea. Retinoids are also used for enhancing desquamation and augmenting the effects of peels with which they are combined. Jessner's and TCA peels are typically used for more advanced photoaging changes including wrinkles. Caution is recommended with more aggressive superficial chemical peels such as TCA 20% and multi-layer Jessner's peels in darker Fitzpatrick skin types (IV–VI), due to their greater risk of PIH; and with patients that have facial erythema and skin sensitivity due to the risk of exacerbating these conditions.

Alternative Therapies

Microdermabrasion is similar to superficial chemical peels in terms of the depth of resurfacing, and is a reasonable alternative treatment for skin rejuvenation. Microdermabrasion has some advantages over chemical peels such as greater control over the depth of exfoliation, less discomfort, and no postprocedure skin flaking or peeling. However, microdermabrasion equipment is more costly than chemical peels. Dermaplaning uses a specialized scalpel blade that is gently scraped across the skin for exfoliation. Successful outcomes with this type of treatment is highly dependent on clinician expertise, although it is a low cost option.

More aggressive skin resurfacing procedures such as medium-depth chemical peels, dermabrasion and laser resurfacing offer significantly greater reduction of wrinkles and improvements in photodamaged skin. However, these more aggressive resurfacing procedures require longer recovery times and have significantly increased risks of complications.

Superficial chemical peels will not improve deep wrinkles related to volume loss and hyperdynamic musculature, which instead respond to treatment with dermal fillers and botulinum toxin, respectively.

Chemical Peel Handling and Storage

Regardless of the type of chemical peel, all products require attentive handling and storage. Lids must be secured and peel containers kept out of direct sunlight and extreme temperatures. A current materials safety data sheet (MSDS) is kept on hand for every peel used which can be obtained from peel manufacturers.

Advantages of Superficial Chemical Peels

- Inexpensive
- Appropriate for all Fitzpatrick skin types
- Multiple conditions treated simultaneously
- Epidermal and dermal improvements
- Appropriate for use on the body

Disadvantages of Superficial Chemical Peels

- Typically require multiple treatments to achieve benefits
- Cannot remove scars, only lessen their appearance

Contraindications

- Allergy to chemical peel constituents
- Aspirin allergy (for salicylic acid peels)
- Pregnancy or nursing
- Active infection or open wound in the treatment area (e.g., herpes simplex, impetigo, and cellulitis)
- Keloidal or hypertrophic scarring
- Melanoma (or lesions suspected for melanoma), basal cell or squamous cell carcinoma in the treatment area
- Dermatoses (e.g., vitiligo, psoriasis, and atopic dermatitis) in the treatment area
- Impaired healing (e.g., due to immunosuppression)
- Skin atrophy (e.g., chronic oral steroid use or genetic syndromes such as Ehlers–Danlos syndrome)
- Bleeding abnormality (e.g., thrombocytopenia)
- Uncontrolled systemic condition
- Deep chemical peel, dermabrasion, or radiation therapy in the treatment area in the preceding 6 months
- Isotretinoin (Accutane) use within the preceeding 6 months
- Excessive laxity and deep skin folds
- Insufficient sun protection (including tanning bed use) pre and postprocedure
- Unrealistic expectations
- Body dysmorphic disorder

Indications and contraindications for each specific chemical peel product are also provided by manufacturers, and providers are advised to follow these for the specific product used.

Equipment

- Headband
- Towel to drape the patient
- Non-sterile gloves

- Eye protection for the patient (adhesive eye pads, goggles, or moist gauze)
- Small bowl for water
- Small ceramic bowl for chemical peel
- Battery operated, handheld fans with soft blades
- 4×4 non-woven gauze
- 2×2 non-woven gauze
- Cotton-tipped applicators (for petrolatum)
- Petrolatum
- Saline eye wash
- Cream facial cleanser (e.g., Creamy Cleanser by PCA SKIN or Gentle Cleanser by SkinCeuticals)
- Alpha hydroxy acid facial cleanser (e.g., Purifying Cleanser by SkinCeuticals or Facial Wash Oily/Problem by PCA SKIN)
- Microbead scrub (e.g., Micro Exfoliating Scrub by SkinCeuticals or Gentle Exfoliant by PCA SKIN)
- Astringent toner (e.g., Equalizing Toner by SkinCeuticals or Smoothing Toner by PCA SKIN) or ethanol 70%
- Chemical peel product(s)
- Topical steroid creams: low potency (hydrocortisone 0.5–2.5%), medium potency (e.g., triamcinolone 0.1%), and high potency (e.g., triamcinolone 0.5%)
- Moisturizer that is soothing and non-occlusive (e.g., Epidermal Repair by SkinCeuticals or ReBalance by PCA SKIN)
- Broad-spectrum sunscreen of SPF 30 or greater containing zinc oxide or titanium dioxide (e.g., Daily Physical Defense SPF 30 by SkinMedica or Weightless Protection SPF 45 by PCA SKIN)

Figure 9 shows a typical tray set-up used for a chemical peel procedure.

Preprocedure Checklist

- Review the patient's medical and cosmetic history (a sample Patient Intake Form is shown in Appendix 2).

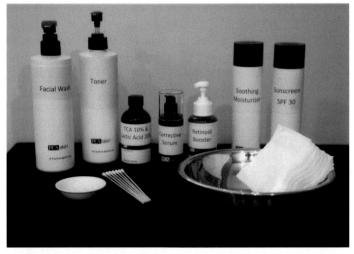

FIGURE 9 ● Equipment set-up for chemical peel procedure. (Courtesy of PCA SKIN)

- Perform an aesthetic consultation (see Introduction and Foundation Concepts, Consultation section).
- Examine the treatment area and document the patient's Fitzpatrick skin type, Glogau score, and the presence of wrinkles, acne, scars, benign vascular or pigmented lesions, oiliness/dryness, and other skin conditions (a sample Skin Analysis Form is shown in Appendix 3).
- Obtain informed consent (see Introduction and Foundation Concepts) (a sample Consent Form is shown in Appendix 4, Consent for Skin Care Treatments).
- Pretreatment photographs are recommended (see Introduction and Foundation Concepts).
- A broad-spectrum sunscreen of SPF 30 or greater that contains zinc oxide or titanium dioxide.
- Two weeks prior to the procedure, advise patients to discontinue tanning and direct sun exposure and avoid for the duration of treatments.
- One to two weeks prior to treatment, advise patients to discontinue products containing high strength AHAs (e.g., glycolic and lactic acids) and prescription retinoids (e.g., Retin A, Renova, and Differin).
- Two days prior to the procedure, start a prophylactic antiviral medication (e.g., acyclovir 400 mg or valacyclovir 500 mg, 1 tablet 2 times per day) for patients with a history of herpes simplex or varicella in or around the treatment area, and continue for 3 days postprocedure.
- The day of the procedure, advise patients to wash the treatment area and remove any facial jewelry and contact lenses.
- A sample preprocedure instruction handout is provided in Appendix 5, Before and After Instructions for Skin Care Treatments.

Preprocedure Skin Care Products

Preparation of the skin prior to chemical peeling using a topical product regimen can enhance peel effects, facilitate postprocedure healing, and reduce the risks of complications. Topical products are typically begun 4–6 weeks preceding the chemical peel and consist of a retinoid, sunscreen, antioxidant, and moisturizer. The Topical Product Regimen for Photoaged Skin can also serve as the preprocedure regimen (see Topical Skin Care Products section). In patients with darker Fitzpatrick skin types (IV–VI) or a predisposition to hyperpigmentation, a lightening agent such as hydroquinone (2–6%) may also be used to help reduce the risk of postprocedure PIH.

Preprocedure retinoid use prepares the skin by decreasing stratum corneum thickness, which ultimately allows for a more even application and uniformity of peel penetration. A prescription retinoid (e.g., retinoic acid) or a non-prescription retinoid (e.g., retinol) may be used. While there is evidence in the literature regarding use of preprocedure prescription strength retinoids, the associated dermatitis can limit their use. Retinol is typically well tolerated by most patients; however, there is limited data supporting non-prescription strength retinoids preprocedure. Topical prescription retinoids are discontinued 1–2 weeks prior to a peel to allow for epidermal healing, and help ensure that the skin is intact at the time of the peel procedure. Chemical peels applied to skin which is not intact can penetrate deeper than intended and may be associated with negative outcomes.

Patch Testing

A "patch test" may be performed prior to a chemical peel procedure to identify potential allergic reaction or adverse response to a specific peel product. Patients with a history of multiple allergies or sensitivities to preservatives and/or fragrances may have an increased risk of allergic reaction. Patch test sites are located discretely near the treatment area, behind the ear for example, or on the dorsum of the forearm. The skin is prepped as usual for peeling, and the desired peel applied, timed, and neutralized if indicated. The site is evaluated 3 days after placement and the test is deemed positive if any of the following are present: excessive erythema, urticaria, vesiculation (i.e., epidermolysis), report of excessive pruritis or pain, or other unusual response. The date, location, and products used in the patch test and description of response are recorded in the chart. If a patch test is positive, the specific chemical peel that was tested is avoided. A negative patch test is reassuring and the treatment may be performed with the tested peel. However, a negative patch test does not ensure that an allergic reaction or adverse response will not occur at the time of treatment with the tested peel.

Anesthesia

Preprocedure anesthesia is typically not required with superficial chemical peels.

Steps for Performing a Chemical Peel Procedure

The main steps for a chemical peel procedure are listed below (and shown in Fig. 10):

1. Preparation (position, drape, cleanse and degrease skin, apply eye protection, and apply petrolatum) (Fig. 11)
2. Chemical peel application (Fig. 12)
3. Termination (Fig. 13)
4. Boost (optional)
5. Topical product application

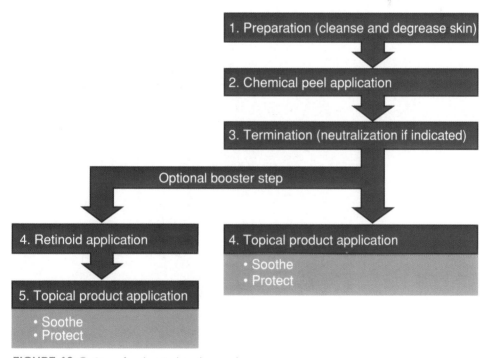

FIGURE 10 ● Steps for chemical peel procedure.

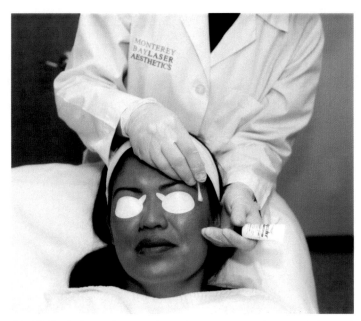

FIGURE 11 ● Application of petrolatum to areas of potential chemical peel pooling. (Courtesy of Rebecca Small, MD)

Chemical peel application and termination vary with different peeling agents and methods for specific peels are outlined in the following chemical peel chapters. Providers are encouraged to follow manufacturer instructions for the specific peel being used.

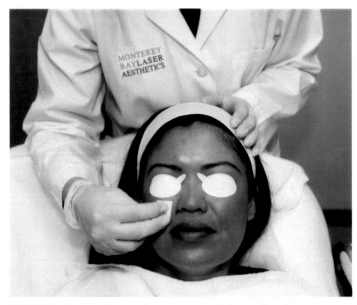

FIGURE 12 ● Technique for application of chemical peel using gauze. (Courtesy of Rebecca Small, MD)

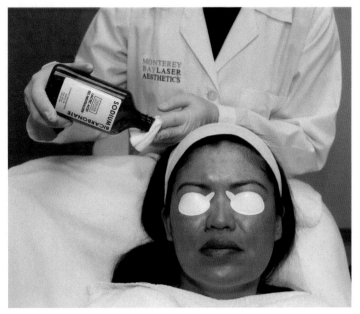

FIGURE 13 ● Neutralization of chemical peel. (Courtesy of Rebecca Small, MD)

Overview of Chemical Peel Procedure

- Skin is prepared prior to peel application using products to cleanse and degrease the skin. Two main skin preparation methods are recommended:
  - **Basic skin prep,** consists of a gentle cleanser, followed by a hydroxy acid cleanser and an astringent toner to degrease the skin.
  - **Intense skin prep,** consists of a gentle cleanser followed by a hydroxy acid cleanser which can be followed by a microbead scrub to remove surface debris, and either an astringent toner or ethanol to degrease the skin. The intense prep helps ensure even application and enhance peel penetration.
- The Chemical Peel Safety Zone is the area within which a chemical peel can most safely be applied to the face (Fig. 14). This region includes the full face outside the eye orbits (above the eyebrows and 2–3 mm below the inferior eyelash margin) and excludes the lips.
- Chemical peels are typically thin liquids that have a tendency to pool in skin folds which can increase the depth of penetration. Common areas of pooling include oral commissures, marionette lines, nasolabial folds particularly at the ala, and lateral canthal creases. Application of petrolatum to these areas as a barrier to protect them from overtreatment is recommended (Figs. 11 and 14).
- Establishing a systematic method for applying chemical peels whereby the provider applies a consistent amount of peel product uniformly with even pressure to the treatment area is very important. Once the provider is a 'constant' without significant variation, other procedural factors such as the number of peel layers can be modified to change treatment intensity.
- Dividing the face into four quadrants aids in applying the peel in a systematic manner (Fig. 15). The peel is applied to the least reactive areas first, such as the forehead, and to the more sensitive areas, such as the medial face last. Figure 16 shows the

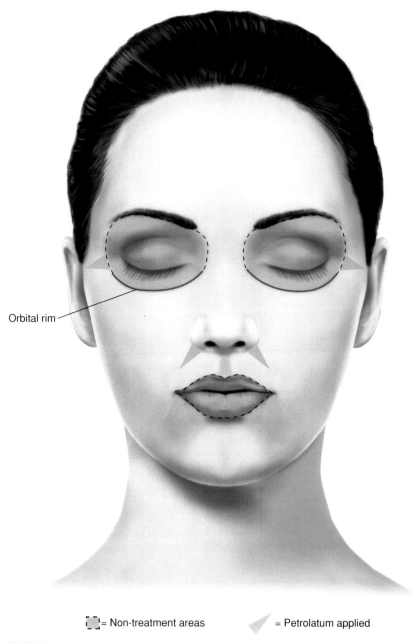

Orbital rim

⬚ = Non-treatment areas   ◢ = Petrolatum applied

FIGURE 14 ● Chemical Peel Safety Zone.

sequence for applying a chemical peel to the face. Chemical peel is applied first to the forehead and then the cheeks. This is followed by application to the medial face starting with the nose, upper lip, and then the chin.

- There are a variety of chemical peel applicators available for applying chemical peels including non-woven gauze (also referred to as cotton squares or gauze sponges), brushes and cotton tipped applicators. Non-woven gauze is the preferred applicator used by the authors. Brushes and cotton-tipped applicators tend to pick up more product and offer less control.

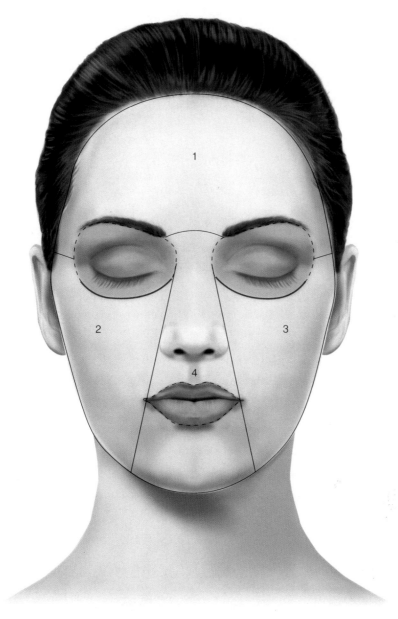

= Non-treatment areas

FIGURE 15 ● Facial quadrants.

- Saturation of the gauze applicator can be performed in several ways, two of which are outlined below. Again, consistency is ultimately more important than the type of applicator chosen or saturation method.
  - **Saturate a 2 × 2 non-woven gauze** with chemical peel solution by placing a dry gauze into a ceramic bowl, and using a dropper, dispense the amount indicated by the manufacturer into the ceramic bowl. Fold the gauze into quarters and squeeze excess acid drops from the gauze into the bowl.
  - Alternatively, **dampen a 4 × 4 non-woven gauze** with chemical peel solution by folding a gauze into quarters and inverting the peel solution bottle onto the gauze, using the number of inversions indicated by the manufacturer.

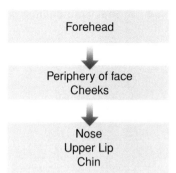

FIGURE 16 ● Sequence for chemical peel application to the face.

• Chemical peel is applied to each facial quadrant using one of the methods shown in Figure 17. Use firm even pressure when sweeping the gauze across the skin.
  • **Quadrant 1, forehead.** Sweep the gauze from the eyebrow up to hairline. Reapply chemical peel solution to the gauze.
  • **Quadrant 2, cheek.** Sweep the gauze from the temple to the jaw line on one side of the face. The cheek can be covered using either horizontal sweeps from medial to lateral (Fig. 17A) or from superior to inferior (Fig. 17B). Reapply the chemical peel solution to the gauze.
  • **Quadrant 3, cheek.** Repeat for the contralateral cheek. Do not reapply chemical peel solution to the gauze.
  • **Quadrant 4, medial face.** Sweep the gauze down the dorsum of the nose, along each nasal sidewall, above the upper lip and then across the chin.

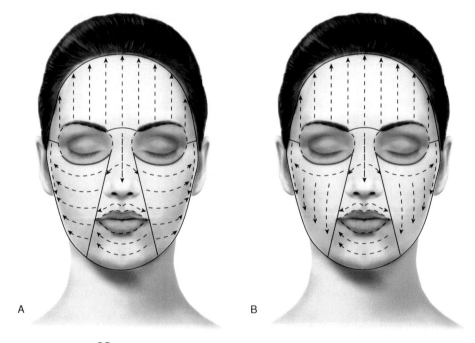

A   B

░ = Non-treatment areas   - - ➔ = Chemical peel application

FIGURE 17 ● Directional guide for applying chemical peel to the face using two methods (**A** and **B**).

- **Feather the edge of the treatment** area with chemical peel by lightly sweeping the gauze 1 cm below the jaw line. This helps avoid a possible line of demarcation between treated and untreated skin.
- Patient's discomfort is assessed during and after peel application using a verbal scale from 1 to 10. Discomfort up to 5 out of 10 is typically acceptable. Tingling, itching, burning and stinging sensations are commonly reported which usually peak within a few minutes of application and then subside. Discomfort of 6 or greater indicates that the peel procedure should be terminated (with neutralization if indicated), any residual peel product removed from the face, and the patient's skin cooled.
- Some chemical peels (e.g., Jessner's peel and TCA) are applied in layers, where a layer is a defined as complete coverage of the treatment area with a single application of chemical peel. Multiple layers increase the quantity of product and hence, the depth of penetration. The skin is observed for a period of time (usually 4–7 minutes) for visible clinical endpoints after each layer. If endpoints are not reached, additional layers may be applied. Each subsequent layer is applied by sweeping the gauze perpendicular to the prior layer to help ensure complete coverage of the treatment area.
- The skin is observed throughout the procedure for desirable and undesirable clinical endpoints which are described below.
  - **Desirable clinical endpoints** for superficial peels depend on the agent used. In most cases mild erythema is the desired endpoint. For TCA, level I frosting visible as patchy whitening with erythema of the skin is the desired endpoint. Peels with salicylic acid, including Jessner's peel, typically form a fine white precipitate that is also a desired clinical endpoint. Table 1 summarizes clinical endpoints for superficial chemical peel agents and they are also reviewed in the individual peel chapters of this book.
  - **Undesirable clinical endpoints** include excessive patient discomfort with pain greater than 6 out of 10; blistering (vesiculation) which is indicative of epidermolysis; "frosting" or whitening of the skin for certain peels (see Table 1). Note that frosting or whitening is a desirable endpoint with salicylic acid and

TABLE 1

Superficial Chemical Peels: Key Properties

Chemical Peel	Neutralization Required	Skin Whitening Desired	Discomfort	Desquamation
Alpha hydroxy acids	Yes	No	++	Inconsistent
Salicylic acid	No	Yes, pseudofrost	++	Yes
Trichloroacetic acid	No	Yes, frost	+++	Yes
Jessner's peel	No	Yes, pseudofrost	++	Yes
Other self-neutralizing blended peels	No	Yes, pseudofrost[a]	+	Yes
Retinoids	No	No	+	Yes

Note: Salicylic acid and Jessner's peels usually form a pseudofrost which is crystallization of the acid rather than true frosting, which is coagulation of epidermal proteins and keratinocytes seen with TCA.

[a]Other self-neutralizing blended peels have a variety of constituent acids. Those with salicylic acid can form a pseudofrost.

+, mild; ++, moderate; +++, intense.

TCA, but **not** with AHAs. Whitening or graying of the skin indicates overtreatment with AHAs.

- The chemical peel procedure is terminated if/when:
  - Desired clinical endpoints are achieved.
  - Desired number of minutes for peeling has been reached (if the peel is a timed procedure).
  - Undesired endpoints occur.
- Most superficial peels such as TCA, retinoids, salicylic acid, and Jessner's peels do not require neutralization and the peel is simply left on the skin. Certain peeling agents, such as glycolic acid, require neutralization to terminate the activity of the acid through application of water or a sodium bicarbonate solution (Table 1).
- Peels that form a white precipitate on the skin (such as salicylic acid and Jessner's peels) may have the precipitate wiped off with dry gauze. True frosting (as seen with TCA) does not wipe off.
- Retinoic acid and non-prescription retinoid (e.g., retinol) peels can be applied on top of the primary chemical peel as a booster to increase cell turnover and speed up the desquamation process. Providers are encouraged to follow manufacturer instructions for using a booster retinoid peel with the primary peel, as the intensity of the overall treatment is increased when these peels are combined.
- Some peel manufacturers recommend application of corrective products immediately following a peel which target specific conditions such as hyperpigmentation and dehydration. These products are usually thin serum formulations and are applied prior to other soothing products and sunscreen. Providers are encouraged to follow manufacturer instructions for using corrective products immediately after peel application to ensure compatibility of peels and products.

Aftercare

Erythema, dryness, mild edema, and skin sensitivity are common in the first 3–5 days postprocedure. The skin may also feel tighter, texture and wrinkles may appear coarser, and patients may report mild pruritis during this time. Desquamation typically starts on day 3–5 postprocedure and ranges from skin flaking to skin sloughing and peeling. If peeling occurs, it usually starts in the midface proceeding towards the periphery, and can persist up to 2 weeks. Figure 18 shows significant desquamation 3 days (A) and 5 days (B) after a TCA 20% peel. In some cases, flaking or peeling may not occur, particularly in patients whose skin is conditioned (i.e., who regularly exfoliates). Patients may require reassurance that, despite lack of desquamation, the skin has histologic benefits from the peel procedure.

For the 1–2 weeks following treatment, **soothing and hydrating topical products** are used and irritating ingredients such as AHAs or retinoids are avoided. An example of a postpeel regimen would include daily use of a gentle cleanser, broad-spectrum sunscreen of SPF 30 or greater containing zinc oxide or titanium dioxide during the day, and a non-occlusive moisturizer in the evening (see Skin Care Products for Pre and Postprocedure in the Topical Skin Care Products section). If **erythema** is marked immediately after treatment, hydrocortisone (0.5% to 2.5%) may be applied twice daily until erythema resolves. This is particularly important for patients with darker skin types (IV–VI) to reduce the risk of PIH. **Makeup** may be worn 24 hours after the procedure and mineral make-up is preferable (e.g., by Jane Iredale or ColorScience). **Strict sun (and tanning bed) avoidance** for 2 weeks postprocedure is advised as well as the use of other sun protective measures

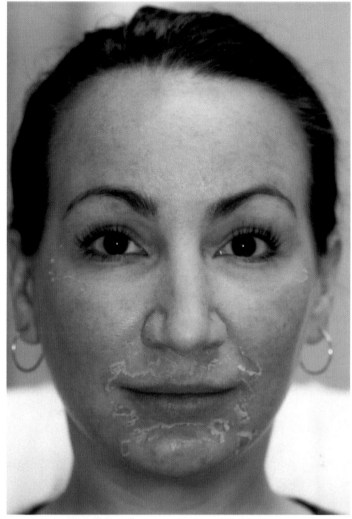

FIGURE 18A ● Desquamation 3 days after a TCA 20% peel. (Courtesy of Rebecca Small, MD) (*continued*)

such as a wide-brimmed hat. Patients are instructed to follow-up if they notice prolonged erythema for 5 days or more, severe pruritis, discomfort, pain, crusting, drainage or other signs or symptoms that deviate from the usual postprocedure course. **Regular skin care products,** such as those used in the Topical Product Regimen discussed in the Topical Skin Care Products section, may be resumed once the skin is no longer irritated or peeling, usually 1–2 weeks postprocedure. An example of a patient postprocedure handout is provided in Appendix 5, Before and After Instructions for Skin Care Treatments.

Common Follow-Ups and Management

- **Excessive dryness** during the posttreatment period can be managed with reapplication of sunscreen in the daytime and substitution of an occlusive moisturizer such as Aquaphor or Primacy in the evening until dryness resolves.
- **Lack of peeling or flaking** does not indicate that a peel was histologically or clinically ineffective and patients may require reassurance regarding this point.

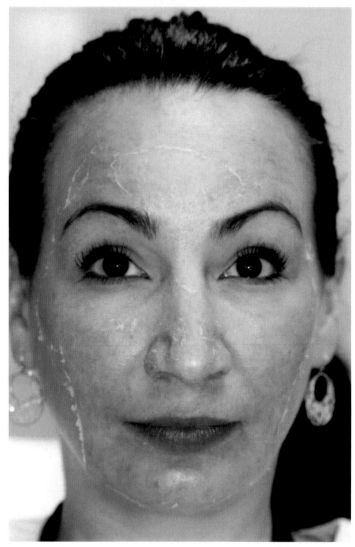

FIGURE 18B ● Desquamation 5 days after a TCA 20% peel. (Courtesy of Rebecca Small, MD)

Results

Improvements in skin texture and brightness may be observed with a single treatment. However, a series of six chemical peels are usually necessary to achieve more marked improvements in skin smoothness, reduction of hyperpigmentation, fine lines, oiliness, and acne. Results can be further enhanced by combining peels with microdermabrasion and topical home care products.

Figure 19 shows a patient with UV-induced hyperpigmentation before (A) and after (B) one treatment with a modified Jessner's peel containing lactic acid 14%, salicylic acid 14% and kojic acid 3%, pH 1.5–1.9. Home care products included daily use of kojic acid and azelaic acid lightening agents (Pigment Gel by PCA SKIN) and a broad-spectrum sunscreen of SPF 30.

Figure 20 shows a patient with photoaging including laxity and fine lines before (A) and after (B) five self-neutralizing blended peels containing TCA 10% and lactic

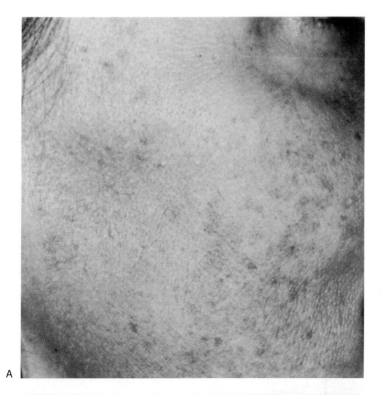

A

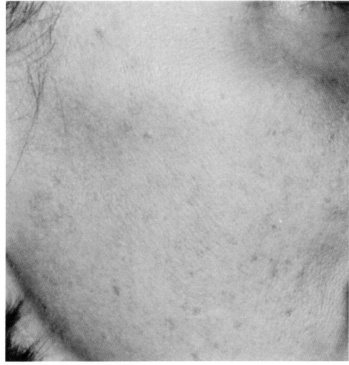

B

FIGURE 19 ● Photodamaged skin with hyperpigmentation before **(A)** and after **(B)** one treatment of a modified Jessner's peel containing lactic acid 14%, salicylic acid 14%, and kojic acid 3% (PCA Peel). (Courtesy of PCA SKIN)

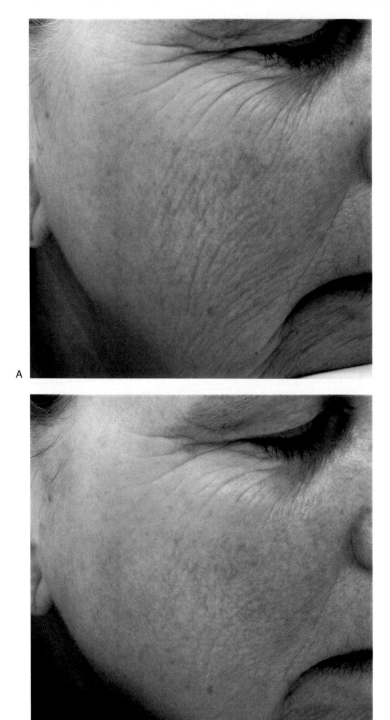

FIGURE 20 ● Photodamaged skin with laxity and fine lines before **(A)** and after **(B)** five treatments of a blended chemical peel containing TCA 10% with lactic acid 20% and a retinol 10% booster peel (Ultra Peel I and Ultra Peel II). (Courtesy of PCA SKIN)

acid 20%, pH 0.6–1; followed by a booster peel of retinol 10%, pH 3.7–4.1. Home care products included daily use of acetyl hexapeptide-8 for skin texture (ExLinea Peptide Smoothing Serum by PCA SKIN), 15% L-ascorbic acid antioxidant (C-Strength 15% with 5% Vitamin E by PCA SKIN), evening moisturizer, and a broad-spectrum sunscreen of SPF 30.

Figure 21 shows a patient with photoaging including fine lines, laxity, coarse pores and mottled pigmentation before (A) and after (B) a progressive chemical peel series of six treatments including two microdermabrasions, lactic acid 45%, TCA 6% with lactic acid 12% and retinol 10% booster, TCA 10% with lactic acid 20% and TCA 20% peels. Home care products included daily use of growth factor for texture (TNS Recovery Complex by SkinMedica) 10% L-ascorbic acid antioxidant (CE Ferulic by SkinCeuticals), hydroquinone 4% for hyperpigmentation (Clear by Obagi), and a broad-spectrum sunscreen of SPF 30 (Ultimate UV Defense by SkinCeuticals).

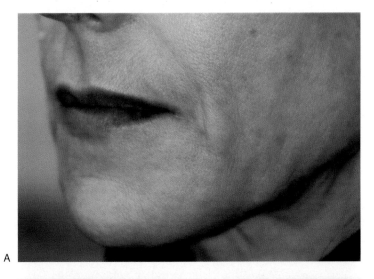

A

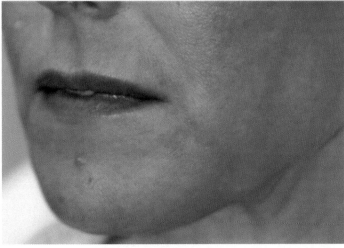

B

FIGURE 21 ● Photodamaged skin with fine lines, laxity, and coarse pores before **(A)** and after **(B)** a progressive chemical peel series including two microdermabrasions, lactic acid 45% (Circadia), TCA 6% with lactic acid 12% and retinoid 10% booster (Sensi Peel and Ultra Peel II by PCA SKIN), TCA 10% with lactic acid 20% (Ultra Peel Forte by PCA SKIN) and a TCA 20% peel (Rhonda Allison). (Courtesy of Rebecca Small, MD)

Learning the Techniques

Providers are encouraged to develop a systematic method for chemical peel application by initially treating staff and friends. In addition, receiving a chemical peel oneself can further provider's understanding of the sensations associated with chemical peel application (e.g., stinging or burning), the sense of relief provided with fanning and postpeel product application, the posttreatment experience of skin tightness, flaking or peeling, and the clinical benefits.

It is advisable to acquire one or two very superficial peel products (see Fig. 2 for superficial peeling agents) and develop a comfort level with those specific products first. Providers should be familiar with the clinical endpoints, typical patient responses, desquamation, and the clinical effects associated with those peels. As procedural proficiency is gained, providers may choose to add a retinoid booster and more aggressive superficial peel products such as TCA 20% to their peel cabinet.

Non-facial Treatment Areas

The skin on the body differs from facial skin as it has fewer pilosebaceous units, which are the sites of re-epithelialization and sebum production. Therefore, non-facial skin is relatively drier, repairs more slowly, has less dramatic improvements with treatments, and is more prone to complications compared to the face. Gentle hydrating peels such as lactic acid and blended peels are commonly used in non-facial areas, particularly for the delicate skin of the anterior neck and chest (décolletage).

Chemical peel application is limited to not more than 25% of the body at any one time. Over-exposure to certain peeling agents, such as salicylic acid, has the potential for systemic toxicity. In addition, peeling a large surface area can be associated with excessive discomfort and postprocedure skin care can be challenging. Total body surface area (TBSA) for different body regions is listed below in Table 2.

Different parts of the body are subject to a variety of skin conditions. Acne is common on the back, hyperpigmentation on the arms, legs and chest, and keratosis pilaris on the upper arms and thighs. Glycolic, lactic and trichloroacetic acid peels are commonly

TABLE 2

Surface Area for Adult Body Regions

Body Region	Total Body Surface Area (%)
Anterior head	4.5
Posterior head	4.5
Anterior torso	18.0
Posterior torso	18.0
Anterior leg (unilateral)	9.0
Posterior leg (unilateral)	9.0
Anterior arm (unilateral)	4.5
Posterior arm (unilateral)	4.5
Genitalia/perineum	1.0

used in non-facial areas for the above conditions. Posttreatment care is the same for peels in non-facial areas and includes protection with a broad-spectrum sunscreen and hydrating topical products.

Progressive Peeling

Progressive peeling refers to increasing the intensity of chemical peels over time. A series of six treatments is typically performed where the depth of resurfacing is progressively increased through the use of very superficial peels in the beginning and superficial peels at the end of the series. This escalation of intensity allows the patient to become acquainted with the experience of peeling gradually, to safely gauge the skin's response to particular peels early on in the series, and helps ensure patient adherence to postprocedure instructions with use of appropriate home care products. As the series progresses, skin becomes more conditioned as the stratum corneum is thinned and leveled, and towards the end of the treatment series more intense and effective peels may be safely performed to help achieve maximal results.

The initial treatment in a series is performed using a very superficial peel, such as glycolic acid, or a microdermabrasion. The subsequent visit typically utilizes the same peeling agent, but the intensity of the treatment is increased. The intensity of a given peel treatment can be increased in several possible ways depending on the acid used, such as increasing the time of application or the numbers of layers applied. For example, if the initial treatment is performed using a glycolic acid peel with a low percentage such as 20% for a short time such as 3 minutes, the time of application for the same peel may be increased to 5–7 minutes at the subsequent visit to intensify the treatment. An alternate example utilizing self-neutralizing blended peels, such as TCA 6% with lactic acid 12%, might start with 1–2 layers on the first visit and at the subsequent visit, the number of layers for the same peel might be increased to three to four. The goal is to continue increasing treatment intensity at each subsequent visit, based in the patient's skin reactivity and tolerance to each procedure. Later in the series, treatments can be intensified by adding a retinoid booster peel on top of the primary peel or by utilizing microdermabrasion as part of skin preparation prior to chemical peel application. Preprocedure exfoliation with microdermabrasion allows for more even and deeper acid penetration. It is advisable to use established manufacturer protocols when combining these two exfoliation modalities as peel characteristics can be altered by removal of the stratum corneum barrier with microdermabrasion. The final treatment in a series may utilize more aggressive superficial peels, such as multi-layer Jessner's peel or TCA 20%. Methods for intensifying of a given peel treatment are discussed in the individual peel chapters of this book (see Intensifying Subsequent Treatments in individual peel chapters).

Selection of peels in a treatment series is guided by the patient's Fitzpatrick skin type and the presenting skin condition. Patients with higher Fitzpatrick skin types (IV–VI) usually require more gentle treatments than patients with lighter skin types (I–III) due to their greater risk of pigmentary changes such as PIH. Below are examples of progressive chemical peel series that may be used to treat photoaging in light and dark Fitzpatrick skin types (Table 3). Many alternative peels are equally appropriate. Examples of progressive chemical peel series that may be used to treat facial erythema (sensitive and rosacea skin), acne and hyperpigmentation are reviewed below in Notes on Specific Lesions and Conditions.

TABLE 3

Progressive Chemical Peel Treatments for Photoaging

	Chemical Peels (Peel Brand Name, Manufacturer)	
Visit	Fitzpatrick I–III	Fitzpatrick IV–VI
1	Glycolic acid 20% with lactic acid 10% 1–3 minutes (Gel Peel GL, SkinCeuticals) or Microdermabrasion	Lactic acid 35% (Circadia) or Microdermabrasion
2	Glycolic acid 35%, 3–5 minutes (NeoStrata)	Salicylic acid 20% (Micropeel Plus 20, SkinCeuticals)
3	TCA 6% with lactic acid 12% 1–3 layers (Sensi Peel, PCA SKIN)	Salicylic acid 30% (Micropeel Plus 30, SkinCeuticals)
4	TCA 10% with lactic acid 20% 1–3 layers (Ultra Peel I, PCA SKIN)	TCA 10% with salicylic acid 20% 1–3 layers (TCA/Salicylic acid, Rhonda Allison)
5	TCA 10% with lactic acid 20% 3 to 5 layers, Plus retinol 10% (Ultra Peel, PCA SKIN), (Ultra Peel II, PCA SKIN)	TCA 10% with salicylic acid 20% 3–5 layers (TCA/Salicylic acid, Rhonda Allison)
6	TCA 20% 1–3 layers (Rhonda Allison)	TCA 15% with salicylic 15% and lactic acid 15%, Plus retinol 10% (Salicylic Solution, Rhonda Allison), (Ultra Peel II, PCA SKIN)

Treatment Intervals

Treatment intervals for peels vary from 2–4 weeks during a series of six treatments, and the interval is determined by the treatment intensity and sensitivity of the patient's skin. **Very superficial peels** or microdermabrasion are commonly performed at the beginning of a series and treatment intervals are usually every **2 weeks**, as the skin recovers rapidly from these treatments. More intense superficial peels performed later in the series, are associated with a greater degree of exfoliation and require more time for re-epithelialization. **Superficial chemical peels** are typically performed every **4 weeks**. After the last peel in a series, such as a TCA 20% peel or a multilayer Jessner's peel, it is advisable to allow a rest period of 2 months. When patients resume skin care treatments, it is advisable to start with very superficial peels or microdermabrasion in the initial visits, and progress to more intense superficial peels over the course of the series.

Complications and Management

- Pain
- Prolonged erythema
- Hyperpigmentation
- Hypopigmentation
- Infection (e.g., acne, impetigo, candidiasis or activation of herpes simplex)
- Milia
- Deeper than intended resurfacing
- Vesiculation (epidermolysis) and crusting
- Allergic reactions including urticaria, papules, and the remote possibility of severe reactions such as anaphylaxis

- Scarring and textural changes
- Salicylism with salicylic acid (very rare)

The risk of complications from chemical peels is primarily related to the depth of skin resurfacing. Superficial chemical peels, which penetrate to the epidermis and possibly the upper papillary dermis, have a low risk of complications. Transient hyperpigmentation in response to prolonged erythema is one of the most common complications encountered. Deeper peels, which can penetrate to the papillary and reticular dermis, have greater potential for severe complications such as scarring and permanent pigmentary changes such as hypopigmentation.

Pain is usually present only at the time of chemical peel application and is typically reported as mild to moderate discomfort. Complaints of postprocedure pain are uncommon and evaluation is advisable, particularly to assess for infection.

Erythema postprocedure is expected and the duration depends on the inherent reactivity of the patient's skin and the depth of resurfacing. Most erythema following superficial peels resolves spontaneously within a few hours, and occasionally lasts up to a few days. This mild erythema can be treated with over-the-counter corticosteroid creams (e.g., hydrocortisone 1%) or topical products containing anti-inflammatory ingredients (e.g., evening primrose oil and bisabolol). Erythema lasting more than 5 days is considered prolonged and can be treated with either a medium potency (triamcinolone 0.1%) or low potency topical steroid cream (hydrocortisone 0.5%–2.5%) twice daily for 3–5 days or until erythema resolves. Sun avoidance is very important postpeel especially when erythema is present, and in patients with darker Fitzpatrick skin types (IV–VI), to reduce the risk of PIH. Patients with severe cases of **erythematous skin conditions** such as telangiectasias, rosacea and Poikiloderma of Civatte are at risk for exacerbation and prolonged erythema with overly aggressive peel treatments. **Contact dermatitis** due to the peel itself, or more often due to one of the postprocedure products, is also a possible cause of prolonged erythema. It is typically associated with pruritis, and may be managed by discontinuing the offending product and application of topical steroids as described above. Resorcinol, a component of Jessner's peels, can be associated with contact dermatitis. **Infection** is also a consideration with prolonged erythema, especially if associated with tenderness (see below).

Hyperpigmentation is one of the most commonly encountered complications with superficial chemical peels and usually occurs in the setting of overly aggressive peeling in patients with a predisposition to hyperpigmentation, and often inadequate sun protection immediately postprocedure. Figure 22 shows a patient with hyperpigmentation in the marionette lines 1 month after receiving a Jessner's chemical peel (6 layers) who did not have petrolatum applied to marionette lines, which is an area of potential chemical peel pooling. Figure 23 shows more profound postinflammatory hyperpigmentation following a glycolic acid 70% peel. Hyperpigmentation can be treated with over-the-counter lightening agents (e.g., hydroquinone 2% or cosmeceutical brightening agents such as kojic, lactic and azelaic acids) or prescription medications (e.g., hydroquinone 4%–8%). Most postinflammatory hyperpigmentation due to superficial peels resolves, but in rare instances it may be permanent. In addition, resolution of PIH in higher Fitzpatrick skin types (IV–VI) can be slow, taking up to 6 months or more. Hyperpigmentation risk increases with sun exposure, the use of hormones, and other photosensitizing medications.

Hypopigmentation is rare with superficial peels. The potential for hypopigmentation is also directly correlated with the intensity of the peel applied. For example, deep phenol

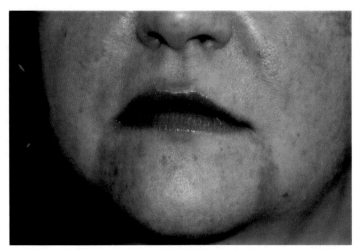

FIGURE 22 ● Postinflammatory hyperpigmentation in the marionette lines 1 month after a Jessner's peel (6 layers) without protective application of petrolatum to areas of pooling. (Courtesy of Rebecca Small, MD)

peels can cause hypopigmentation even in lower Fitzpatrick skin types. Repigmentation can improve hypopigmentation in some cases; however, it is often permanent.

Infections are rare with superficial peels and require treatment specific to the infection. **Acne exacerbations** may be treated with oral medications, such as doxycycline or minocycline, as topical acne therapies can be irritating to skin postpeel. **Herpes simplex** activation may occur despite appropriate pretreatment with an anti-viral medication. These

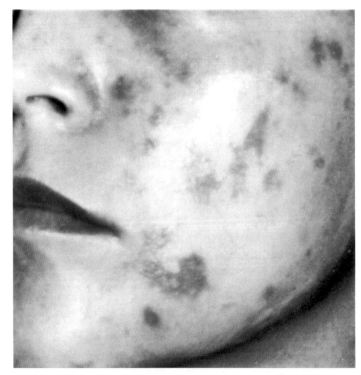

FIGURE 23 ● Postinflammatory hyperpigmentation after a 70% glycolic acid peel. (Courtesy of PCA SKIN)

vesicular lesions are most commonly seen on the vermillion border or lateral nose, but can occur at any previous site of HSV infection. Due to the risk of spread with non-intact skin, aggressive treatment should be employed, usually with an anti-viral medication that is different from the prophylactic medication used (e.g. vancyclovir 1 gm twice or maximally 3 times per day for 7 days until the skin is fully re-epithelialized). **Cutaneous candidiasis** often presents as bright red patches with small surrounding erythematous macules occurring in the perioral area and pruritis. Topical antifungals or oral fluconazole may be used (e.g., 150 mg daily for 3 days). Staphylococcus and streptococcus are common pathogens for **bacterial infections** and require treatment with appropriate antibiotics (e.g., initial empiric coverage may include doxycycline 100 mg twice daily or cephalexin 500 mg 4 times daily, and if methicillin resistant staphylococcus aureus or anaerobes are suspected, clindamycin 300 mg 4 times daily). It is advisable to culture infections if there is a question regarding the diagnosis prior to initiating therapy.

Milia are tiny 1–2 mm white papules that result from occlusion of sebaceous glands. Petrolatum-based products (e.g., Aquaphor) used to hydrate skin can occlude sebaceous glands and contribute to milia formation. Milia do not usually resolve spontaneously and require lancing with a 20 gauge needle and extraction (e.g., gentle squeezing with cotton-tipped applicators).

Deeper than intended resurfacing can occur with superficial peels if the skin is not intact at the time of peel application. The skin barrier can be disrupted by topical retinoid products, overly aggressive exfoliation (e.g., daily home use of exfoliating sponges or scrubs, aggressive microdermabrasion), shaving, frequent abrasion with a beard or moustache, acne pustules, and seborrheic or atopic dermatitis. Pooling of peel solutions can also be associated with deeper than intended penetration. At the time of treatment undesirable clinical endpoints may be evident, such as level II or above frosting. Figure 24 shows deeper than intended peel penetration with level II frosting (A) from application of 1 layer of a Jessner's peel in a patient using retinoic acid immediately preprocedure, and delayed healing (B). **Vesiculation (epidermolysis),** evident as small vesicles at the time of peel application, is due to deep tissue penetration and is extremely uncommon with superficial peels. Glycolic acid peels formulated with high concentrations and very low pHs (pH < 2) have an increased risk of epidermolysis. Use of an occlusive ointment (e.g., Aquaphor or Bacitracin) and a bandage is recommended for hydration during the healing process until re-epithelialization occurs.

Allergic reactions to chemical peels are rare. The most commonly encountered allergic reaction is urticaria, which responds to oral antihistamines (e.g., cetirizine 10 mg) and medium potency (triamcinolone 0.1%) or high potency (triamcinolone 0.5%) topical steroid creams may be used. There is a remote risk of severe allergic reactions, such as bronchospasm and anaphylaxis, necessitating emergency care. Salicylic acid containing peels have the highest risk of allergic response and should not be used with patients that have an allergy to aspirin.

Scarring is extremely rare with superficial peels. The risk of scarring is increased with medium or deep peels, laser resurfacing, dermabrasion, isotretinoin use, radiation therapy or facial surgery within the preceding 6 months; connective tissue disease (e.g. Ehlers-Danlos syndrome), and other factors which impair wound healing such as smoking and chronic disease. Scarring is also more common in patients with a history of abnormal healing such as keloid formation, and if postprocedure infection occurs. Tissue in which scarring is imminent usually appears as bright red patches with textural changes. Treatment with high potency topical steroids (e.g., Cordran tape) and pulsed dye lasers can be helpful in reducing scarring.

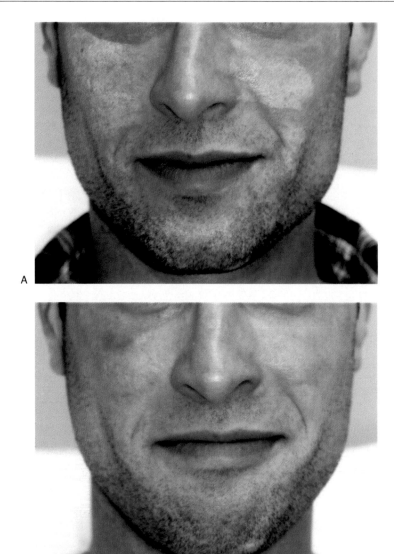

FIGURE 24 ● Deeper than intended peel penetration in a patient using retinoic acid showing level II frosting **(A)** and delayed healing day 9 **(B)** on the right cheek after application of 1 layer of a Jessner's peel. (Courtesy of Rebecca Small, MD)

Systemic toxicity due to over-exposure to peeling agents can occur. Cases of salicylate toxicity, or salicylism, with signs of nausea, disorientation and tinnitus have been reported in patients receiving salicylic acid peels on non-intact skin. Chemical peel treatment of large body surfaces (e.g., more than 25% total body surface area) are also avoided to reduce the risk of chemical peel toxicity.

Notes on Specific Lesions and Conditions

Below are examples of chemical peel series that can be used to treat common aesthetic skin conditions including facial erythema (Table 4), acne (Table 5), and hyperpigmentation (Table 6), in patients with light (I–III) and dark (IV–VI) Fitzpatrick skin types. Many alternative selections of peels are equally appropriate.

TABLE 4

Progressive Chemical Peel Treatments for Facial Erythema: Sensitive Skin and Rosacea in Fitzpatrick Skin Types I–VI

Visit	Chemical Peels (Peel Brand Name, Manufacturer)
1	Lactic acid 35% (Circadia)
2	Lactic acid 45% (Circadia)
3	TCA 6% with lactic acid 12% (Sensi Peel, PCA SKIN)
4	TCA 6% with lactic acid 12%, plus retinoid 10% (Sensi Peel and Ultra Peel II, PCA SKIN)
5	TCA 10% with lactic 20% (Ultra Peel I, PCA SKIN)
6	TCA 10% with lactic 20%, plus retinoid 10% (Ultra Peel I and Ultra Peel II, PCA SKIN)

TABLE 5

Progressive Chemical Peel Treatments for Acne

	Chemical Peels (Peel Brand Name, Manufacturer)	
Visit	Fitzpatrick I–III	Fitzpatrick IV–VI
1	Salicylic acid 20% with mandelic acid 10% (Gel Peel SM, SkinCeuticals) or Microdermabrasion	Salicylic acid 20% with mandelic acid 10% (Gel Peel SM, SkinCeuticals) or Microdermabrasion
2	Salicylic acid 20% (Micropeel Plus 20, SkinCeuticals)	Salicylic acid 20% (Micropeel Plus 20, SkinCeuticals)
3	Salicylic acid 30% (Micropeel Plus 30, SkinCeuticals)	Salicylic acid 30% (Micropeel Plus 30, SkinCeuticals)
4	Jessner's 1–3 layers (Jessner's peel, Global Skin Solutions)	TCA 10% with salicylic acid 20% 1–3 layers (TCA/Salicylic acid, Rhonda Allison)
5	Jessner's 3–5 layers, plus retinoid 10% (Jessner's peel, Global Skin Solutions), (Ultra Peel II, PCA SKIN)	TCA 10% with salicylic acid 20% 3–5 layers (TCA/Salicylic acid, Rhonda Allison)
6	Jessner's 3–5 layers, plus retinoic acid 0.3% (Jessner's peel, Global Skin Solutions), (tretinoin, University Specialty Pharmacy)	TCA 15% with salicylic acid 15% and lactic acid 15%, plus retinoid 10% 1–3 layers (Salicylic Solution, Rhonda Allison), (Ultra Peel II by PCA SKIN)

TABLE 6

Progressive Chemical peel Treatments for Hyperpigmentation

| Visit | Chemical Peels (Peel Brand Name, Manufacturer) | |
	Fitzpatrick I–III	Fitzpatrick IV–VI
1	Salicylic acid 20% with mandelic acid 10% (Gel Peel SM, SkinCeuticals) or Microdermabrasion	Salicylic acid 20% with mandelic acid 10% (Gel Peel SM, SkinCeuticals) or Microdermabrasion
2	Salicylic acid 20% (Micropeel Plus 20, SkinCeuticals)	Salicylic acid 20% (Micropeel Plus 20, SkinCeuticals)
3	Salicylic acid 30% (Micropeel Plus 30, SkinCeuticals)	Salicylic acid 30% (Micropeel Plus 30, SkinCeuticals)
4	Enhanced Jessner's[a] 1–3 layers (PCA Peel with HQ and Resorcinol, PCA SKIN)	Modified Jessner's[b] 1–3 layers (PCA Peel with HQ, PCA SKIN)
5	Enhanced Jessner's[a] 3–5 layers (PCA Peel with HQ and Resorcinol, PCA SKIN)	Modified Jessner's[b] 3–5 layers (PCA Peel with HQ, PCA SKIN)
6	Enhanced Jessner's[a] 3–5 layers, plus retinoic acid 0.3% (PCA Peel with HQ and Resorcinol, PCA SKIN), (tretinoin, University Specialty Pharmacy)	Modified Jessner's[b] 3–5 layers, plus retinoid 10% (PCA Peel with HQ and Ultra Peel II, PCA SKIN)

[a]Enhanced Jessner's = Lactic acid 14%, salicylic acid 14%, resorcinol 14%, kojic acid 3%, and hydroquinone 2%.
[b]Modified Jessner's = Lactic acid 14%, salicylic acid 14%, kojic acid 3%, and hydroquinone 2%.

Combining Aesthetic Treatments

Enhanced results for treatment of photoaged skin, and other skin conditions such as hyperpigmentation and acne, can be achieved by combining chemical peels with the other skin care treatments discussed throughout this practical guide: microdermabrasion and daily skin care products. Chemical peels can also be safely combined with other minimally invasive aesthetic procedures such as laser and intense pulsed light, or injectable procedures to enhance rejuvenation results (see Combination Therapies in the Introduction and Foundation Concepts section for additional information about combination treatments).

Reimbursement and Financial Considerations

Chemical peels can be obtained from skin care product companies or medical suppliers (see Appendix 8, Chemical Peel and Topical Product Supply Sources). A 2 oz. bottle of a chemical peel can be purchased for approximately $50–$80 which yields about 20 peels. Patient fees for chemical peels vary by geographic region and range from $65–$450 based on the peel procedure. The more aggressive higher strength superficial peels tend to have higher fees (e.g., Jessner's and pure TCA peels). Some insurance companies cover chemical peel treatments for indications such as acne and actinic keratosis, however, most do not. Chemical peels are often performed and charged for as a series of six treatments. Committing to a treatment series helps achieve the best possible results and ensure high patient and provider satisfaction.

CTP Codes

- 15788   Chemical peel, facial; epidermal
- 15789   Chemical peel, facial; dermal
- 15792   Chemical peel, nonfacial; epidermal
- 15793   Chemical peel, nonfacial; dermal

ICD-9 Codes

- 706.1   Acne
- 695.3   Rosacea
- 702.0   Actinic Keratosis
- 709.00   Dyschromia, unspecified

Chapter 2

Alpha Hydroxy Acid Peel: Glycolic Acid

Chemical Peel	Neutralization Required	Clinical Endpoint	Whitening Desired	Discomfort	Desquamation
Glycolic acid (GA)	Yes	Mild erythema	No	++	Inconsistent

+ Mild, ++ Moderate, +++ Intense.

This chapter describes how to perform a superficial chemical peel with glycolic acid (GA), one of the most commonly used alpha hydroxy acids (AHAs). It is also applicable for blended peels containing GA. For procedural information on blended peels containing other AHAs, see the chapter on Other Self-Neutralizing Blended Peels.

Chemical Peel Steps

1. Preparation position, drape, cleanse and degrease skin, apply eye protection and petrolatum
2. Chemical peel application
3. Termination
4. Boost (optional)
5. Topical product application

Chemical Peel Selection, Contraindications, Equipment, Preprocedure Checklist, Preprocedure Skin Care Products, Patch Testing, Steps for Performing a Chemical Peel Procedure, Overview of Chemical Peel Procedure

See Chemical Peel Introduction and Foundation Concepts section.

Primary Factors Modified to Increase Peel Depth

- Application time
- Chemical peel concentration

Many other factors can increase GA peel depth and they are outlined in the Factors Influencing the Depth of Chemical Peel Penetration, Chemical Peel Introduction and Foundation Concepts section.

Other Practical Considerations with AHA Peels

- **Formulations.** AHA peels are usually clear, colorless solutions or gels. Strengths of pure GA products used for superficial peels are typically 20–70%. Strengths of pure LA products used for superficial peels are typically 20–50%. Strengths of GA or LA used in blended peels are typically 10–20%.
- **Patch testing.** Patch testing is recommended for all chemical peels (see Patch Testing, Chemical Peel Introduction and Foundation Concepts section, for testing methodology and interpretation).

Performing a Superficial Alpha Hydroxy Acid Chemical Peel Using Glycolic Acid 20%

The following procedure uses glycolic acid 20% (by NeoStrata) as an example of an alpha hydroxy acid chemical peel. Techniques vary for products from different manufacturers, and providers are advised to familiarize themselves with protocols for the specific agent used and to follow manufacturer's instructions.

Preparation: Position, Drape, Cleanse and Degrease Skin, Apply Eye Protection and Petrolatum

1. Setup all products necessary for the procedure within arms' reach.
   - GA is neutralized using water or a sodium bicarbonate solution (5–15%). Saturate a stack of 4×4 gauze with the neutralizer by placing the dry gauze into a small bowl and pouring the neutralizing agent into the bowl.
2. Position the patient supine on the treatment table.
3. Using a headband or surgical cap, secure patient's hair away from the face.
4. Drape a towel across the neck and chest to protect patient's clothing.
5. Apply gentle cleanser to the face with gloved hands and use fingertips to rub the cleanser in small circular motions. Remove using 4×4 gauze moistened with water.
6. Cleanse the face a second time with a hydroxy acid cleanser using the method above.
7. Degrease the skin with an astringent toner using 2×2 gauze. The same application technique that will be used for the peeling solution can also be used to degrease the skin so as to reinforce the application method (see step 13 below). Allow the skin to dry.
8. Examine the skin again and limit treatment areas if necessary.
   - Acne lesions may be treated, but it is advisable to avoid treatment of all other areas with non-intact skin.

9. Cover the patient's eyes with disposable adhesive pads or moistened gauze for protection.

10. Apply petrolatum sparingly to areas of potential pooling using a cotton-tipped applicator including the lateral canthal creases, nasolabial folds particularly at the ala, oral commissures, and marionette lines.

Chemical Peel Application

11. Select the appropriate peel and desired applicator. Glycolic acid 20% peel with a 2 × 2 non-woven gauze applicator are used here.

12. Saturate the 2 × 2 gauze with the chemical peel solution by placing one dry gauze into a ceramic bowl and, using a dropper, dispense the amount indicated by the manufacturer into the ceramic bowl. Fold the gauze into quarters and squeeze excess acid drops from the gauze into the bowl. Dry gloved hands on a towel.

13. Apply the GA peel evenly to the face with the 2 × 2 gauze using the established pattern for peel application outlined in the Chemical Peel Procedure Overview, Chemical Peel Introduction and Foundation Concepts section.
    - **Quadrant 1, forehead.** Using firm even pressure, sweep the gauze from the eyebrow up to hairline.
    - **Quadrant 2, cheek.** Re-saturate the gauze with chemical peel solution in the ceramic bowl as described above. Sweep the gauze from the temple to the jawline on one side of the face. The cheek can be covered using horizontal sweeps either from medial to lateral or from superior to inferior.
    - **Quadrant 3, cheek.** Re-saturate the gauze with chemical peel solution in the ceramic bowl as described above. Repeat for the contralateral cheek.
    - **Quadrant 4, medial face.** Do not re-saturate the gauze with peel solution. Sweep the gauze down the dorsum of the nose, along each nasal sidewall, above the upper lip and then across the chin.
    - **Feather the edge of the treatment** area with chemical peel by lightly sweeping the gauze 1 cm below the jawline. This helps avoid a possible line of demarcation between treated and untreated skin.
    - Attempt to complete application within 30 seconds so as not to increase the treatment time in areas where first applied.
    - **Open bottles or soaked applicators should never be passed over the patient's eyes.** If peel solution enters the patient's eyes, copiously flush the eye immediately with normal saline solution or water.
    - If deep wrinkles are present, stretch the skin while applying the peel to reduce the potential for peel solution to pool in wrinkles.

14. After 1 layer of the peel has been applied to the treatment area begin timing the procedure.
    - Each patient's tolerance will vary but, ideally, the peel solution should remain on the skin for 3 minutes.

15. Provide the patient with a handheld fan. Self-fanning reduces discomfort and serves as a distraction.

16. Communicate with the patient regarding any sensations or discomfort they may be feeling using a pain scale of 1 to 10.
    - Tingling, itching, burning, or stinging sensations are common and typically peak 2–3 minutes after application and then subside.
    - Discomfort up to a 5 or 6 out of 10 is acceptable.

17. Observe the skin throughout treatment for desirable and undesirable clinical endpoints.

> Desirable clinical endpoints for alpha hydroxy acid chemical peels include
>
> • **Mild erythema**
>
> Undesirable clinical endpoints for alpha hydroxy acid chemical peels include
>
> • **Blistering/vesiculation** which is indicative of epidermolysis
> • **Blanching or whitening** of the skin
> • **Excessive patient discomfort** with pain greater than 6 out of 10, or overly irritating sensations

18. Acne lesions may frost due to deeper peel penetration. Frosting will not wipe off with gauze.

Termination

19. The chemical peel procedure is terminated if/when
    • Desired clinical endpoint of mild erythema is visible, or
    • Chemical peel is applied for 3 minutes (even if mild erythema is not observed), or
    • Undesired endpoints occur including blistering/vesiculation, whitening of the skin or excessive patient discomfort
20. GA peel activity is terminated through neutralization using water or a sodium bicarbonate solution (10–15%). Apply neutralizer briskly to the face by wiping 4×4 gauze saturated with neutralizer from the center of the face to the periphery. Repeat application of the neutralizer using freshly saturated gauze 2–3 times or more.
    • Areas of greatest discomfort are neutralized first.
    • Patients often report a transient increase in heat/discomfort initially with the application of neutralizer.
21. Wrapped ice packs or cold moistened towels may be applied at the end of the peel procedure for patient comfort. Fanning may be continued as desired for comfort.

Boost (Optional)

22. **Retinoid peels** can be applied after the GA peel has been terminated, if there are no undesirable endpoints, to intensify the treatment and speed the desquamation process.
    • It is advisable to first perform the GA peel procedure without a retinoid booster to ensure tolerability to the primary peel.
    • Dry the skin by fanning or with gauze before applying the retinoid booster peel. See Retinoid Peel chapter for information on applying booster peels.
    • Providers are encouraged to follow manufacturer recommendations regarding using booster retinoid peels with the primary peel to confirm the appropriateness of combining these peels and ensure compatibility.

Topical Product Application

23. **Soothe.** Assess the skin for the degree of erythema and apply soothing topical products as outlined below.
    - **Moderate–severe erythema:** apply a high potency steroid cream (e.g., triamcinolone 0.5%), avoiding the periocular area.
    - **Moderate erythema:** apply a medium potency steroid cream (e.g., triamcinolone 0.1%), avoiding the periocular area.
    - **Mild erythema:** apply either a low potency steroid cream (e.g., hydrocortisone 0.5% to 2.5%) or a soothing moisturizer (e.g., SkinCeuticals Epidermal Repair or PCA SKIN's Calming Balm).
24. **Protect.** Apply a **broad-spectrum sunscreen** of SPF 30 or higher containing zinc oxide or titanium dioxide at the conclusion of treatment to protect the skin from UV exposure (e.g., products by Skin Medica, Solar Protection, SkinCeuticals or PCA SKIN).

Aftercare

- Patients requiring topical steroids immediately after treatment will benefit from inclusion of a topical steroid in their postprocedure home care regimen to further reduce erythema and hence, the risk of postinflammatory hyperpigmentation.
- Acne lesions that have frosted may form a crust 1–2 days after treatment. This is managed with daily application of bacitracin until resolved.

See Aftercare, Chemical Peel Introduction and Foundation Concepts section for aftercare instructions.

Treatment Intervals, and Complications and Management

See Chemical Peel Introduction and Foundation Concepts section.

Progressive Peeling: Increasing Intensity of Subsequent Treatments

Glycolic acid peel treatments can be intensified at subsequent visits by increasing the depth of peel penetration in several possible ways:

- **Application time.** Extending the time that the peel remains on the skin (i.e., the application time) is usually the first step in intensifying GA treatments. For example, a GA 20% peel which was initially applied for 3 minutes, may be applied for 3–5 minutes at a subsequent visit to increase the treatment intensity.
- **Peel concentration.** Using a chemical peel product with a higher concentration can intensify GA treatments. For example, after an initial treatment with a GA 20% peel, the subsequent treatment may be performed with the next higher acid concentration such as GA 50%. If that is tolerated, consider using GA 70% at a subsequent visit.
- **Boost.** An additional retinoid peel may be applied after the primary GA peel, to increase treatment intensity and enhance desquamation. For example, after a treatment with a GA 20% peel, the subsequent treatment may be intensified by applying a non-prescription retinoid such as retinol 10% at the booster step of the peel process. At a subsequent visit, the treatment may be further intensified by applying retinol 15% with lactic acid 10%. If the higher strength retinol is tolerated, a prescription-strength retinoid such as retinoic acid 0.3% may be used as the booster at a subsequent visit (for Fitzpatrick skin types I–III).

- **Skin preparation.** For initial peel treatments, skin is commonly prepared prior to peel application using the basic prep described in the Preparation section of this chapter. At subsequent treatments, a more intense prep can be used to enhance peel penetration and intensify the treatment (see Overview of Chemical Peel Procedure, Chemical Peel Introduction and Foundation Concepts section).
- **Microdermabrasion.** Microdermabrasion may be performed prior to the application of a GA peel to remove the stratum corneum barrier and allow for more even and increased peel penetration. For example, two passes with a microdermabrasion using a mild–moderate abrasive element with a mild–moderate vacuum setting may be performed immediately prior to a GA peel to intensify the treatment. Using established manufacturer protocols when combining these two exfoliation modalities is recommended, as peel characteristics and depth of penetration can be significantly increased by the lack of the stratum corneum.
- **Modify one treatment parameter at a time** (e.g., application time, peel concentration, boost, skin preparation, or pretreatment exfoliation) to increase treatment intensity in as safe and controlled a manner as possible. Usually, the time of the procedure is the first variable to be increased while the acid concentration remains the same. At the next visit the concentration is increased while the time is unchanged, and so on.
- **Treatment intensity** may be increased at a subsequent visit only if a patient has demonstrated tolerability to a given peel procedure. Skin is dynamic and variables outside of the providers control may also change, such as patients' preprocedure product regimen, all of which can alter the skin and its response to chemical peel treatments. Therefore, it may not be possible to increase treatment intensity at every visit.
- **Progressive peeling protocols** for photoaged skin (see Progressive Peeling) and other common aesthetic skin conditions such as sensitive skin, acne and hyperpigmentation (see Notes on Specific Lesions and Conditions) are reviewed in the Chemical Peel Introduction and Foundation Concepts section.

Financial Considerations and Coding

Charges for AHA peels vary by geographic region and typically range from $65 to $150 per treatment. Chemical peels are often performed and charged as a series of six treatments to help achieve the best possible results and ensure high patient and provider satisfaction.

Supply Sources

See Appendix 8, Chemical Peel and Topical Product Supply Sources.

Chapter 3

Beta Hydroxy Acid Peel: Salicylic Acid

Chemical Peel	Neutralization Required	Clinical Endpoint	Whitening Desired	Discomfort	Desquamation
Salicylic acid (SA)	No	Mild erythema	Yes, pseudofrost	++	Inconsistent

+ Mild, ++ Moderate, +++ Intense.

This chapter describes how to perform a superficial chemical peel with salicylic acid (SA), the most commonly used beta hydroxy acid (BHA). For procedural information on blended peels containing BHAs, see the chapter on Other Self-Neutralizing Blended Peels.

Chemical Peel Steps

1. Preparation position, drape, cleanse and degrease skin, apply eye protection and petrolatum
2. Chemical peel application
3. Termination
4. Boost (optional)
5. Topical product application

Chemical Peel Selection, Contraindications, Equipment, Preprocedure Checklist, Preprocedure Skin Care Products, Patch Testing, Steps for Performing a Chemical Peel Procedure, Overview of Chemical Peel Procedure

See Chemical Peel Introduction and Foundation Concepts section.

Contraindications

- Aspirin allergy

See Chemical Peel Introduction and Foundation Concepts for additional contraindications.

Primary Factors Modified to Increase Peel Depth

- Greater number of layers
- Chemical peel concentration

Increasing the number of layers, where a layer is defined as complete coverage of the treatment area with chemical peel product, deposits a greater quantity of product on the skin and thereby increases the depth of penetration. Many other factors can increase SA peel depth and they are outlined in the Factors Influencing the Depth of Chemical Peel Penetration, Chemical Peel Introduction and Foundation Concepts section.

Other Practical Considerations with BHA Peels

- **Formulations.** BHA peels are usually solutions or gels. Strengths of pure SA products used for superficial peels range from 10% to 30%.
- **Patch testing.** Patch testing is recommended for all chemical peels (see Patch Testing, Chemical Peel Introduction and Foundation Concepts section, for testing methodology and interpretation).
- **Toxicity.** Salicylate toxicity, or salicylism, is extremely rare with SA peel concentrations used for superficial peels. Signs of salicylism include nausea, disorientation, and tinnitus. Application to large body surfaces (e.g., more than 25% of total body surface area, such as the whole back) is avoided to reduce the risk of toxicity (see Table 2, Chemical Peel Introduction and Foundation Concepts section, for body surface areas).

Performing a Superficial Beta Hydroxy Acid Chemical Peel Using Salicylic Acid 20%

The following procedure uses salicylic acid 20% (Micropeel Plus 20 by SkinCeuticals) as an example of a beta hydroxy acid chemical peel. Techniques vary for products from different manufacturers, and providers are advised to familiarize themselves with protocols for the specific agent used and to follow manufacturer's instructions.

Preparation: Position, Drape, Cleanse and Degrease Skin, Apply Eye Protection and Petrolatum

1. Setup all products necessary for the procedure within arms' reach.
2. Position the patient supine on the treatment table.
3. Using a headband or surgical cap, secure patient's hair away from the face.
4. Drape a towel across the neck and chest to protect patient's clothing.
5. Apply gentle cleanser to the face with gloved hands and use fingertips to rub the cleanser in small circular motions. Remove using 4×4 gauze moistened with water.
6. Cleanse the face a second time with a hydroxy acid cleanser using the method above.

7. Degrease the skin using an astringent toner with 2 × 2 gauze. The same application technique that will be used with the peeling solution can also be used to degrease the skin so as to reinforce the application method (see step 13 below). Allow the skin to dry.
8. Examine the skin again and limit treatment areas if necessary.
   • Acne lesions may be treated, but it is advisable to avoid treatment of all other areas with non-intact skin.
9. Cover the patient's eyes with disposable adhesive pads or moistened gauze for protection.
10. Apply petrolatum sparingly to areas of potential pooling using a cotton-tipped applicator including the lateral canthal creases, nasolabial folds particularly at the ala, oral commissures, and marionette lines.

Chemical Peel Application

11. Select the appropriate peel and desired applicator. A 2 × 2 non-woven gauze applicator is used here.
12. Saturate the 2 × 2 gauze with the chemical peel solution by placing one dry gauze into a ceramic bowl and, using a dropper, dispense the amount indicated by the manufacturer into the ceramic bowl. Fold the gauze into quarters and squeeze excess acid drops from the gauze into the bowl. Dry gloved hands on a towel.
13. Apply the SA peel evenly to the face with the 2 × 2 gauze using the established pattern for peel application outlined in the Chemical Peel Procedure Overview, Chemical Peel Introduction and Foundation Concepts section.
    • **Quadrant 1, forehead.** Using firm even pressure, sweep the gauze from the eyebrow up to hairline.
    • **Quadrant 2, cheek.** Re-saturate the gauze with chemical peel solution in the ceramic bowl as described above. Sweep the gauze from the temple to the jawline on one side of the face. The cheek can be covered using horizontal sweeps either from medial to lateral or from superior to inferior.
    • **Quadrant 3, cheek.** Re-saturate the gauze with chemical peel solution in the ceramic bowl as described above. Repeat for the contralateral cheek.
    • **Quadrant 4, medial face.** Do not re-saturate the gauze with peel solution. Sweep the gauze down the dorsum of the nose, along each nasal sidewall, above the upper lip, and then across the chin.
    • **Feather the edge of the treatment** area with chemical peel by lightly sweeping the gauze 1 cm below the jawline. This helps avoid a possible line of demarcation between treated and untreated skin.
    • **Open bottles or soaked applicators should never be passed over the patient's eyes.** If the peel solution enters the patient's eyes, copiously flush the eye immediately with normal saline solution or water.
    • If deep wrinkles are present, stretch the skin while applying the peel to reduce the potential for peel solution to pool in wrinkles.
14. After 1 layer of the peel has been applied to the treatment area, begin the timer to monitor the duration of the procedure.
15. Provide the patient with a handheld fan. Self-fanning reduces discomfort and serves as a distraction.

16. Communicate with the patient regarding any sensations or discomfort they may be feeling using a pain scale of 1 to 10.
    - Tingling, itching, burning, or stinging sensations are common and typically peak 2–3 minutes after application, and then subside.
    - Discomfort up to a 5 or 6 out of 10 is acceptable.
17. Observe the skin throughout treatment for desirable and undesirable clinical endpoints.

Desirable clinical endpoints for beta hydroxy acid chemical peels include

- **Mild erythema**
- **White powdery residue ("pseudofrost")**

Undesirable clinical endpoints for beta hydroxy acid chemical peels include

- **Blistering/vesiculation** which is indicative of epidermolysis
- **Excessive patient discomfort** with pain greater than 6 out of 10, or overly irritating sensations

---

18. A white powdery residue typically forms on the skin 1–2 minutes after the first layer of peel is applied, which represents crystallization of SA and is different from frosting seen with TCA. Wait 2–3 minutes to ensure the peel has fully penetrated, and then wipe off the residue with dry gauze.
19. Acne lesions may truly frost due to deeper peel penetration. Frosting will not wipe off with gauze.
20. Apply additional peel layers to the face, for a total of 2–3 layers, using the above technique. The first layer typically provides an anesthetic effect and subsequent layers usually have minimal discomfort. Avoid acne lesions that have frosted.
21. After the last layer is applied, wait 2–3 minutes and then wipe off any powdery residue using dry gauze.

Termination

22. The chemical peel procedure is terminated if/when
    - Desired clinical endpoint of mild erythema is visible, or
    - Undesired endpoints occur including blistering/vesiculation, frosting, or excessive patient discomfort
23. Salicylic acid peels are self-neutralizing and, therefore, do not require application of a neutralizing agent.
24. If undesirable clinical endpoints occur, attempt to remove any excess peel product from the skin using gauze saturated with water. Place a stack of dry 4 × 4 gauze into a small bowl and pour water into the bowl. Using the moistened gauze, briskly wipe the face from the center to the periphery. Repeat using freshly saturated gauze 2–3 times or more. Apply wrapped ice packs or cold moistened towels to the face to reduce discomfort. Patients often report a transient increase in heat/discomfort when water is applied. Fanning may be continued as desired for comfort.

Boost (Optional)

25. **Retinoid peels** can be applied after the SA peel has terminated, if there are no undesirable endpoints, to intensify the treatment and speed the desquamation process.
    - It is advisable to first perform the SA peel procedure without a retinoid booster to ensure tolerability to the primary peel.
    - Dry the skin by fanning or with gauze prior applying the retinoid booster peel. See Retinoid Peel chapter for information on applying booster peels.
    - Providers are encouraged to follow manufacturer instructions for using a booster retinoid peel with the primary peel to confirm the appropriateness of combining these peels and ensure compatibility.

Topical Product Application

26. **Soothe.** Assess the skin for the degree of erythema and apply a soothing topical product as outlined below:
    - **Moderate–severe erythema:** apply a high potency steroid cream (e.g., triamcinolone 0.5%), avoiding the periocular area.
    - **Moderate erythema:** apply a medium potency steroid cream (e.g., triamcinolone 0.1%), avoiding the periocular area.
    - **Mild erythema:** apply either a low potency steroid cream (e.g., hydrocortisone 0.5% to 2.5%) or a soothing moisturizer (e.g., SkinCeuticals Epidermal Repair or PCA SKIN's Calming Balm).
27. **Protect.** Apply a **broad-spectrum sunscreen** of SPF 30 or higher containing zinc oxide or titanium dioxide at the conclusion of treatment to protect the skin from UV exposure (e.g., products by Skin Medica, Solar Protection, SkinCeuticals or PCA SKIN).

Aftercare

- Patients requiring topical steroids immediately after treatment will benefit from inclusion of a topical steroid in their postprocedure home care regimen to further reduce erythema and hence the risk of postinflammatory hyperpigmentation.
- Acne lesions that have frosted may form a crust 1–2 days after treatment. This is managed with daily application of bacitracin until resolved.

See Aftercare, Chemical Peel Introduction and Foundation Concepts section for aftercare instructions.

Treatment Intervals, and Complications and Management

See Chemical Peel Introduction and Foundation Concepts for these sections.

Progressive Peeling: Increasing Intensity of Subsequent Treatments

Salicylic acid peel treatments can be intensified at subsequent visits by increasing the depth of peel penetration in several possible ways:

- **Peel concentration.** Using a chemical peel product with a higher concentration of SA is usually the first step in intensifying SA treatments. For example, after an initial treatment with a SA 20% peel, the subsequent treatment may be performed using the next higher strength of acid such as SA 30%.

- **Boost.** An additional retinoid peel may be applied after the final layer of SA peel, to increase treatment intensity and enhance desquamation. For example, after a treatment with a SA 30% peel, the subsequent treatment may be performed by applying a non-prescription retinoid such as retinol 10% at the booster step of the peel process. At the next visit, the treatment may be further intensified by applying a stronger retinoid such as retinoic acid 0.3% as the booster (for Fitzpatrick skin types I–III).
- **Skin preparation.** For initial peel treatments, skin is commonly prepared prior to peel application using the basic prep described in the Preparation section of this chapter. At subsequent treatments, a more intense prep can be used to enhance peel penetration and intensify the treatment (see Overview of Chemical Peel Procedure, Chemical Peel Introduction and Foundation Concepts section, for skin preparation before peeling).
- **Microdermabrasion.** Microdermabrasion may be performed prior to the application of a SA peel to remove the stratum corneum barrier and allow for more even and increased peel penetration. For example, two passes with a microdermabrasion using a mild–moderate abrasive element with a mild–moderate vacuum setting may be performed immediately prior to a SA peel to intensify the treatment. Using established manufacturer protocols is recommended when combining these two exfoliation modalities as peel characteristics and depth of penetration can be significantly altered by the lack of the stratum corneum.
- **Modify one treatment parameter at a time** (e.g., concentration, boost, skin preparation, or pretreatment exfoliation) to increase treatment intensity in as safe and controlled manner as possible. The peel percentage is usually the first SA variable to be increased. Once the desired percentage is reached, the intensity of the subsequent treatment can be increased either with pretreatment exfoliation (microdermabrasion) or by using a booster peel.
- **Treatment intensity** may be increased at a subsequent visit only if a patient has demonstrated tolerability to a given peel procedure. Skin is dynamic and variables outside of the providers control may also change, such as patients' preprocedure product regimen, all of which can alter the skin and its response to chemical peel treatments. Therefore, it may not be possible to increase treatment intensity at every visit.

Financial Considerations and Coding

Charges for SA peels vary by geographic region and typically range from $65 to $150 per treatment. Chemical peels are often performed and charged as a series of six treatments to help achieve the best possible results and ensure high patient and provider satisfaction.

Supply Sources

See Appendix 8, Chemical Peel and Topical Product Supply Sources.

Chapter 4

Trichloroacetic Acid Peel

Chemical Peel	Neutralization Required	Clinical Endpoint	Whitening Desired	Discomfort	Desquamation
Trichloroacetic acid (TCA)	No	Mild–moderate erythema	Yes, level I frosting	+++	Yes

+ Mild, ++ Moderate, +++ Intense.

This chapter describes how to perform a superficial chemical peel using trichloroacetic acid (TCA). For procedural information on blended peels containing TCA, see the chapter on Other Self-Neutralizing Blended Peels.

Chemical Peel Steps

1. Preparation position, drape, cleanse and degrease skin, apply eye protection and petrolatum
2. Chemical peel application
3. Termination
4. Boost (optional)
5. Topical product application

Chemical Peel Selection

- While superficial peels may be used in all Fitzpatrick skin types (I–VI), caution is recommended when using TCA 20% peels to treat darker skin types (IV–VI) due to their greater risk of pigmentary complications such as postinflammatory hyperpigmentation and hypopigmentation.

See Chemical Peel Introduction and Foundation Concepts for additional information on peel selection.

Chemical Peel Selection, Contraindications, Equipment, Preprocedure Checklist, Preprocedure Skin Care Products, Patch Testing, Steps for Performing a Chemical Peel Procedure, Overview of Chemical Peel Procedure

See Chemical Peel Introduction and Foundation Concepts section.

Primary Factors Modified to Increase Peel Depth

- Greater number of layers
- Chemical peel concentration

Increasing the number of layers, where a layer is defined as complete coverage of the treatment area with chemical peel product, deposits a greater quantity of product on the skin and thereby increases the depth of penetration. Many other factors can increase TCA peel depth and they are outlined in the Factors Influencing the Depth of Chemical Peel Penetration, in the Chemical Peel Introduction and Foundation Concepts section.

Other Practical Considerations with TCA Peels

- **Formulations.** TCA peels are usually solutions. Strengths of pure TCA products used for superficial peels are up to 20%.
- **Patch testing.** Patch testing is recommended for all chemical peels (see Patch Testing, Chemical Peel Introduction and Foundation Concepts section, for testing methodology and interpretation).

Performing a Superficial Chemical Peel Using Trichloroacetic Acid 20%

The following procedure uses TCA 20% (by Rhonda Allison) as an example. Techniques vary for products from different manufacturers, and providers are advised to familiarize themselves with protocols for the specific agent used and to follow manufacturer's instructions.

Preparation: Position, Drape, Cleanse and Degrease Skin, Apply Eye Protection and Petrolatum

1. Setup all products necessary for the procedure within arms' reach.
2. Position the patient supine on the treatment table.
3. Using a headband or surgical cap, secure patient's hair away from the face.
4. Drape a towel across the neck and chest to protect patient's clothing.
5. Apply gentle cleanser to the face with gloved hands and use fingertips to rub the cleanser in small circular motions. Remove using 4×4 gauze moistened with water.
6. Cleanse the face a second time with a hydroxy acid cleanser using the method above.
7. (Optional) Scrub the face with a microbead product using the method above. Use gauze to dry the skin and gently wipe away any remaining microbeads.
8. Degrease the skin using an astringent toner or alcohol with 2×2 gauze. The same application technique that will be used with the peeling solution can also be used

to degrease the skin so as to reinforce the application method (see step 14). Allow the skin to dry.

9. Examine the skin again and limit treatment areas if necessary. It is advisable to avoid treatment of all open lesions (including acne lesions).

10. Cover the patient's eyes with disposable adhesive pads or moistened gauze for protection.

11. Apply petrolatum sparingly to areas of potential pooling using a cotton-tipped applicator including the lateral canthal creases, nasolabial folds particularly at the ala, oral commissures, and marionette lines, as well as acne lesions.

Chemical Peel Application

12. Select the appropriate peel and desired applicator. A 2 × 2 non-woven gauze applicator is used here.

13. Saturate the 2 × 2 gauze with the chemical peel solution by placing a dry gauze into a ceramic bowl and, using a dropper, dispense the amount indicated by the manufacturer into the ceramic bowl. Fold the gauze in quarters and squeeze excess acid drops from the gauze into the bowl. Dry gloved hands on a towel.

14. Apply the TCA peel evenly to the face with the 2 × 2 gauze using the established pattern for peel application outlined in the Chemical Peel Procedure Overview, Chemical Peel Introduction and Foundation Concepts section.

- **Quadrant 1, forehead.** Using firm even pressure, sweep the gauze from the eyebrow up to hairline.
- **Quadrant 2, cheek.** Re-saturate the gauze with chemical peel solution in the ceramic bowl as described above. Sweep the gauze from the temple to the jawline on one side of the face. The cheek can be covered using horizontal sweeps either from medial to lateral or from superior to inferior.
- **Quadrant 3, cheek.** Re-saturate the gauze with chemical peel solution in the ceramic bowl as described above. Repeat for the contralateral cheek.
- **Quadrant 4, medial face.** Do not re-saturate the gauze with peel solution. Sweep the gauze down the dorsum of the nose, along each nasal sidewall, above the upper lip, and then across the chin.
- **Feather the edge of the treatment** area with chemical peel by lightly sweeping the gauze 1 cm below the jawline. This helps avoid a possible line of demarcation between treated and untreated skin.
- **Open bottles or soaked applicators should never be passed over the patient's eyes.** If the peel solution enters the patient's eyes, copiously flush the eye immediately with normal saline solution or water.
- If deep wrinkles are present, stretch the skin while applying the peel to reduce the potential for peel solution to pool in wrinkles.

15. After 1 layer of the peel has been applied to the treatment area, begin the timer to monitor the duration of the procedure.

16. Provide the patient with a handheld fan. Self-fanning reduces discomfort and serves as a distraction.

17. Communicate with the patient regarding any sensations or discomfort they may be feeling using a pain scale of 1 to 10.

- Tingling, burning, or stinging sensations are common and typically peak 2–3 minutes after application, and then subside.
- Discomfort up to a 5 or 6 out of 10 is acceptable.

18. Observe the skin throughout treatment for desirable and undesirable clinical end-
    points.

Desirable clinical endpoints for trichloroacetic acid chemical peels
include

- **Mild–moderate erythema**
- **Level I frosting (faint skin whitening with patchy erythema)**

Undesirable clinical endpoints for trichloroacetic acid chemical peels
include

- **Blistering/vesiculation** which is indicative of epidermolysis
- **Excessive patient discomfort** with pain greater than 6 out of 10, or
  overly irritating sensations

---

19. Wait 2–3 minutes to ensure the peel has fully penetrated. Assess the skin for the
    degree of erythema and overlying white discoloration, referred to as frosting. Frost-
    ing represents coagulation of surface proteins and keratinocytes.
    - Level I frosting, visible as faint skin whitening with patchy erythema, is the
      desired endpoint for superficial TCA peels.
    - Acne lesions often frost due to deeper peel penetration.
20. If frosting is not visible on the face, apply another peel layer to the face using the
    above technique. Each layer increases the depth of penetration.
21. Wait 3–5 minutes and assess the skin. If erythema is mild to moderate and frosting
    is still not apparent, apply a final third layer as described above.

Termination

22. The chemical peel procedure is terminated if/when
    - Desired clinical endpoint of mild to moderate erythema is visible or
    - Level I frosting (faint skin whitening with patchy erythema) or
    - Undesired endpoints occur including blistering/vesiculation, opaque whitening
      of the skin or excessive patient discomfort
23. TCA peels are self-neutralizing and, therefore, do not require application of a
    neutralizing agent.
24. If undesirable clinical endpoints occur, attempt to remove any excess peel
    product from the skin using gauze saturated with water. Place a stack of dry
    4 × 4 gauze into a small bowl and pour water into the bowl. Using the moist-
    ened gauze, briskly wipe the face from the center to the periphery. Repeat using
    freshly saturated gauze, 2–3 times or more. Apply wrapped ice packs or cold
    moistened towels to the face to reduce discomfort. Fanning may be continued
    as desired for comfort.

Boost

- **Retinoid peels** are not typically applied after pure TCA peels such as TCA 20%.

Topical Product Application

25. **Soothe.** Assess the skin for the degree of erythema and apply a soothing topical product as outlined below:
    - **Moderate–severe erythema:** apply a high potency steroid cream (e.g., triamcinolone 0.5%), avoiding the periocular area.
    - **Moderate erythema:** apply a medium potency steroid cream (e.g., triamcinolone 0.1%), avoiding the periocular area.
    - **Mild erythema:** apply either a low potency steroid cream (e.g., hydrocortisone 0.5% to 2.5%) or a soothing moisturizer (e.g., SkinCeuticals Epidermal Repair or PCA SKIN's Calming Balm).
26. **Protect.** Apply a **broad-spectrum sunscreen** of SPF 30 or higher containing zinc oxide or titanium dioxide at the conclusion of treatment to protect the skin from UV exposure (e.g., products by Skin Medica, Solar Protection, SkinCeuticals or PCA SKIN).

Aftercare

- Frosting usually disappears within 1–2 hours and erythema becomes more evident. Desquamation with TCA peels is more significant than with most other superficial peels.
- Patients requiring topical steroids immediately after treatment will benefit from inclusion of a topical steroid in their postprocedure home care regimen to further reduce erythema and hence the risk of postinflammatory hyperpigmentation.

See Aftercare, Chemical Peel Introduction and Foundation Concepts section for aftercare instructions.

Treatment Intervals, and Complications and Management

See Chemical Peel Introduction and Foundation Concepts for these sections.

Progressive Peeling: Increasing Intensity of Subsequent Treatments

Trichloroacetic acid peel treatments can be intensified at subsequent visits by increasing the depth of peel penetration in several possible ways:

- **Peel concentration.** Using a chemical peel product with a higher concentration of TCA increases the depth of penetration and intensifies treatments. For example, after an initial treatment with a TCA 10% peel, the subsequent treatment may be performed using the next higher strength of acid, such as TCA 20%.
- **Number of layers.** Applying more layers is usually the first step in increasing TCA treatment intensity. For example, if a treatment is terminated after 2 layers with a TCA 20% peel, the subsequent treatment using the same peel may have 3–5 layers with the goal of achieving level I frosting.
- **Modify one treatment parameter at a time** (e.g., concentration or number of layers) to increase treatment intensity in as safe and controlled a manner as possible.
- **Treatment intensity** may be increased at a subsequent visit only if a patient has demonstrated tolerability to a given peel procedure. Skin is dynamic and variables outside of the providers control may also change, such as patients' preprocedure product regimen, all of which can alter the skin and its response to chemical peel

treatments. Therefore, it may not be possible to increase treatment intensity at every visit.

Financial Considerations and Coding

Charges for TCA peels vary by geographic region and typically range from $400 to $900 for a pure TCA 20% peel treatment. Pure TCA peels are often used as one of the final treatments in a chemical peel series and may be charged separately or as part of a series of six treatments.

Supply Sources

See Appendix 8, Chemical Peel and Topical Product Supply Sources.

Chapter 5

Jessner's Peel

Chemical Peel	Neutralization Required	Clinical Endpoint	Skin Whitening Desired	Discomfort	Desquamation
Jessner's peel	No	Mild–moderate erythema	Yes, pseudofrost	++	Yes

+ Mild, ++ Moderate, +++ Intense.

This chapter describes how to perform a chemical peel using Jessner's peel, one of the most well known and widely used self-neutralizing blended peels. The standard Jessner's peel formulation contains lactic acid 14%, salicylic acid 14%, and resorcinol 14%.

Chemical Peel Steps

1. Preparation position, drape, cleanse and degrease skin, apply eye protection and petrolatum
2. Chemical peel application
3. Termination
4. Boost (optional)
5. Topical product application

Chemical Peel Selection

- While superficial peels may be used in all Fitzpatrick skin types (I–VI), caution is recommended with multilayer Jessner's peels when treating darker skin types (IV–VI) due to their greater risk of pigmentary complications such as postinflammatory hyperpigmentation and hypopigmentation.

See Chemical Peel Introduction and Foundation Concepts for additional information on peel selection.

Chemical Peel Selection, Contraindications, Equipment, Preprocedure Checklist, Preprocedure Skin Care Products, Patch Testing, Steps for Performing a Chemical Peel Procedure, Overview of Chemical Peel Procedure

See Chemical Peel Introduction and Foundation Concepts section.

Contraindications

- Aspirin allergy

See Chemical Peel Introduction and Foundation Concepts for additional contraindications.

Primary Factors Modified to Increase Peel Depth

- Greater number of layers

Increasing the number of layers, where a layer is defined as complete coverage of the treatment area with chemical peel product, deposits a greater quantity of product on the skin and thereby increases the depth of penetration. Many other factors can increase the depth of Jessner's peels and they are outlined in the Factors Influencing the Depth of Chemical Peel Penetration in the Chemical Peel Introduction and Foundation Concepts section.

Practical Considerations with Jessner's Peels

- **Formulations.** Jessner's peels are usually solutions containing lactic acid 14%, salicylic acid 14%, and resorcinol 14%. Enhanced Jessner's peels are also available which include standard Jessner's ingredients in addition to condition specific ingredients, such as hydroquinone or kojic acid for treatment of hyperpigmentation.
- **Patch testing.** Patch testing is recommended for all chemical peels (see Patch Testing, Chemical Peel Introduction and Foundation Concepts section, for testing methodology and interpretation).
- **Toxicity and adverse reactions.** Resorcinol, a component in the Jessner's peel, is a phenol derivative. When used alone in high concentrations (greater than 50%) resorcinol can be associated with toxicity such as myxedema due to anti-thyroid activity, and methemoglobinemia in children. Resorcinol has been associated with contact dermatitis, visible as erythema and edema, at the concentrations used in Jessner's peels (see Complications and Management, Chemical Peel Introduction and Foundation Concepts section). Salicylate toxicity, or salicylism, is extremely rare with blended peels containing salicylic acid such as Jessner's peel. Signs of salicylism include nausea, disorientation, and tinnitus, and cases have been reported with application of salicylic acid to non-intact skin. Large body surfaces (e.g., more than 25% of total body surface area, such as a whole back) are avoided to reduce the risk of toxicity (see Table 2, Chemical Peel Introduction and Foundation Concepts section, for body surface areas).

Performing a Superficial Jessner's Chemical Peel (Lactic Acid 14%, Salicylic Acid 14%, and Resorcinol 14%)

The following procedure uses a standard Jessner's peel (by Global Skin Solutions) as an example. Techniques vary for products from different manufacturers, and providers are advised to familiarize themselves with protocols for the specific Jessner's peel used and to follow manufacturer's instructions.

Preparation: Position, Drape, Cleanse and Degrease Skin, Apply Eye Protection and Petrolatum

1. Setup all products necessary for the procedure within arms' reach.
2. Position the patient supine on the treatment table.
3. Using a headband or surgical cap, secure patient's hair away from the face.
4. Drape a towel across the neck and chest to protect patient's clothing.
5. Apply gentle cleanser to the face with gloved hands and use fingertips to rub the cleanser in small circular motions. Remove using 4×4 gauze moistened with water.
6. Cleanse the face a second time with a hydroxy acid cleanser using the method above.
7. (Optional) Scrub the face with a microbead product using the method above. Use gauze to dry the skin and gently wipe away any remaining microbeads.
8. Degrease the skin with an astringent toner or alcohol using 2×2 gauze. The same application technique that will be used for the peeling solution can be used to degrease the skin so as to reinforce the application method (see step 14 below). Allow the skin to dry.
9. Examine the skin again and limit treatment areas if necessary.
   - Acne lesions may be treated, but it is advisable to avoid treatment of all other areas with non-intact skin.
10. Cover the patient's eyes with disposable adhesive pads or moistened gauze for protection.
11. Apply petrolatum sparingly to areas of potential pooling using a cotton-tipped applicator including the lateral canthal creases, nasolabial folds particularly at the ala, oral commissures, and marionette lines.

Chemical Peel Application

12. Select the appropriate peel and desired applicator. A 2×2 non-woven gauze applicator is used here.
13. Saturate the 2×2 gauze with the chemical peel solution by placing one dry gauze into a ceramic bowl and, using a dropper, dispense the amount indicated by the manufacturer into the ceramic bowl. Fold the gauze in quarters and squeeze excess acid drops from the gauze into the bowl. Dry gloved hands on a towel.
14. Apply the Jessner's peel evenly to the face with the 2×2 gauze using the established pattern for peel application outlined in the Chemical Peel Procedure Overview, Chemical Peel Introduction and Foundation Concepts section.
    - **Quadrant 1, forehead.** Using firm even pressure, sweep the gauze from the eyebrow up to hairline.
    - **Quadrant 2, cheek.** Re-saturate the gauze with chemical peel solution in the ceramic bowl as described above. Sweep the gauze from the temple the jawline on one side of the face. The cheek can be covered using horizontal sweeps either from medial to lateral or from superior to inferior.
    - **Quadrant 3, cheek.** Re-saturate the gauze with chemical peel solution in the ceramic bowl as described above. Repeat for the contralateral cheek.

- **Quadrant 4, medial face.** Do not re-saturate the gauze with peel solution. Sweep the gauze down the dorsum of the nose, along each nasal sidewall, above the upper lip, and then across the chin.
- **Feather the edge of the treatment** area with chemical peel by lightly sweeping the gauze 1 cm below the jawline. This helps avoid a possible line of demarcation between treated and untreated skin.
- **Open bottles or soaked applicators should never be passed over the patient's eyes.** If peel solution enters the patient's eyes, copiously flush the eye immediately with normal saline solution or water.
- If deep wrinkles are present, stretch the skin while applying the peel to reduce the potential for peel solution to pool in wrinkles.

15. Provide the patient with a handheld fan. Self-fanning reduces discomfort and serves as a distraction.
16. Communicate with the patient regarding any sensations or discomfort they may be feeling using a pain scale of 1 to 10.
    - Tingling, itching, burning, or stinging sensations are common and typically peak 2–3 minutes after application, and gradually subsides over 10 minutes.
    - Discomfort up to a 5 or 6 out of 10 is acceptable.
17. Observe the skin throughout treatment for desirable and undesirable clinical endpoints.

Desirable clinical endpoints for Jessner's peels include

- **Mild erythema**
- **White crystal residue ("pseudofrost")**

Undesirable clinical endpoints for Jessner's peels include

- **Blistering/vesiculation** which is indicative of epidermolysis
- **Excessive patient discomfort** with pain greater than 6 out of 10, or overly irritating sensations

---

18. Once applied, erythema is usually followed by a powdery whitening of the skin due to precipitation of salicylic acid (which represents crystallization of SA and is different from frosting seen with TCA). This white powder residue typically forms on the skin 1–2 minutes after the first layer of peel is applied. Wait 2–3 minutes to ensure the peel has fully penetrated, and then dust off the residue with dry gauze.
19. Acne lesions may truly frost due to deeper peel penetration. Frosting will not wipe off with gauze.
20. Apply additional peel layers to the face, for a total of 2–3 layers using the above technique. The first layer typically provides an anesthetic effect and subsequent layers are usually associated with less discomfort. Avoid acne lesions that have frosted.
21. After the last layer, wait 2–3 minutes and then dust off any white residue using dry gauze.

Termination

22. The chemical peel procedure is terminated if/when
    - Desired clinical endpoint of mild erythema is visible, or
    - Undesired endpoints occur including blistering/vesiculation, frosting, or excessive patient discomfort.

23. Jessner's peels are self-neutralizing and, therefore, do not require application of a neutralizing agent.
24. If undesirable clinical endpoints occur, attempt to remove any excess peel product from the skin using gauze saturated with water. Place a stack of dry 4 × 4 gauze into a small bowl and pour water into the bowl. Using the moistened gauze, briskly wipe the face from the center to the periphery. Repeat using freshly saturated gauze 2–3 times or more. Apply wrapped ice packs or cold moistened towels to the face to reduce discomfort. Fanning may be continued as desired for comfort.

Boost (Optional)

25. **Retinoid peels** can be applied after the Jessner's peel has terminated, if there are no undesirable endpoints, to intensify the treatment and speed the desquamation process
    - It is advisable to first perform the Jessner's peel procedure without a retinoid booster to ensure tolerability to the primary peel.
    - Dry the skin by fanning or with gauze before applying the retinoid booster peel. See Retinoid Peel chapter for information on applying booster peels.
    - Providers are encouraged to follow manufacturer instructions for using a booster retinoid peel with the primary peel to confirm the appropriateness of combining the peels and ensure compatibility.

Topical Product Application

26. **Soothe.** Assess the skin for the degree of erythema and apply a soothing topical product as outlined below:
    - **Moderate–severe erythema:** apply a high potency steroid cream (e.g., triamcinolone 0.5%), avoiding the periocular area.
    - **Moderate erythema:** apply a medium potency steroid cream (e.g., triamcinolone 0.1%), avoiding the periocular area.
    - **Mild erythema:** apply either a low potency steroid cream (e.g., hydrocortisone 0.5% to 2.5%) or a soothing moisturizer (e.g., SkinCeuticals Epidermal Repair or PCA SKIN's Calming Balm).
27. **Protect.** Apply a **broad-spectrum sunscreen** of SPF 30 or higher containing zinc oxide or titanium dioxide at the conclusion of treatment to protect the skin from UV exposure (e.g., products by Skin Medica, Solar Protection, SkinCeuticals or PCA SKIN).

Aftercare

- Patients requiring topical steroids immediately after treatment will benefit from inclusion of a topical steroid in their postprocedure home care regimen to further reduce erythema and hence the risk of postinflammatory hyperpigmentation.
- Acne lesions that have frosted may form a crust 1–2 days after treatment. This is managed with daily application of bacitracin until resolved.

See Aftercare, Chemical Peel Introduction and Foundation Concepts section for aftercare instructions.

Treatment Intervals, and Complications and Management

See Chemical Peel Introduction and Foundation Concepts for these sections.

Progressive Peeling: Increasing Intensity of Subsequent Treatments

Jessner's peels can be intensified at subsequent visits by increasing the depth of peel penetration in several possible ways:

- **Number of layers.** Applying additional layers is usually the first step in increasing treatment intensity with Jessner's peels. For example, if a treatment is terminated after 2 layers with a Jessner's peel, the goal for the subsequent treatment may be 3–5 layers.
- **Boost.** An additional retinoid peel may be applied after the final layer of a Jessner's peel to increase treatment intensity and enhance desquamation. For example, after a treatment with 5 layers of a Jessner's peel, the subsequent treatment may be performed by applying a non-prescription retinoid such as retinol 10% at the booster step of the peel process. At the next visit, the treatment may be further intensified by applying a stronger retinoid such as retinoic acid 0.3% as the booster (for Fitzpatrick skin types I–III).
- **Microdermabrasion pretreatment.** Microdermabrasion may be performed prior to the application of a Jessner's peel to remove the stratum corneum barrier and allow for more even and increased peel penetration. For example, two passes with a microdermabrasion using a mild–moderate abrasive element with mild–moderate vacuum setting may be performed immediately prior to a Jessner's peel to intensify the treatment. Using established manufacturer protocols is recommended when combining these two exfoliation modalities as peel characteristics and depth of penetration can be significantly altered by the lack of the stratum corneum.
- **Modify one treatment parameter at a time** (e.g., number of layers, boost, or pretreatment exfoliation) to increase treatment intensity in as safe and controlled manner as possible. Once the desired number of layers is reached, the intensity of the subsequent treatment can be increased either with pretreatment exfoliation (microdermabrasion) or by using a booster peel.
- **Treatment intensity** may be increased at a subsequent visit only if a patient has demonstrated tolerability to a given peel procedure. Skin is dynamic and variables outside of the providers control may also change, such as patients' preprocedure product regimen, all of which can alter the skin and its response to chemical peel treatments. Therefore, it may not be possible to increase treatment intensity at every visit.

Financial Considerations and Coding

Charges for Jessner's peels vary by geographic region and typically range from $110 to $275 per treatment. Chemical peels are often performed and charged as a series of six treatments to help achieve the best possible results and ensure high patient and provider satisfaction.

Supply Sources

See Appendix 8, Chemical Peel and Topical Product Supply Sources.

Chapter 6

Other Self-Neutralizing Blended Peels: Trichloroacetic Acid and Lactic Acid

Chemical Peel	Neutralization Required	Endpoint Desired	Skin Whitening Desired	Discomfort	Desquamation
Self-neutralizing blended peels	No	Mild erythema	Rarely, pseudofrost[a]	+	Yes

+ Mild, ++ Moderate, +++ Intense.

[a]Pseudofrost may form with blended peels containing salicylic acid.

This chapter describes how to perform a superficial chemical peel using a self-neutralizing blended peel containing trichloroacetic acid (TCA) and lactic acid (LA). Methods used for blended peels vary based on the constituents and their formulation. The methods described here are specific to the manufacturer for the example product and differ slightly from those in other chapters of this book with regard to application technique, management of undesirable endpoints, and use of corrective topical products immediately following peel application. Blended peels that require neutralization (e.g., containing glycolic acid) are discussed in the Alpha Hydroxy Acid Peel chapter of this book.

Chemical Peel Steps

1. Preparation position, drape, cleanse and degrease skin, apply eye protection and petrolatum
2. Chemical peel application
3. Termination
4. Boost (optional)
5. Topical product application

Chemical Peel Selection, Contraindications, Equipment, Preprocedure Checklist, Preprocedure Skin Care Products, Patch Testing, Steps for Performing a Chemical Peel Procedure, Overview of Chemical Peel Procedure

See Chemical Peel Introduction and Foundation Concepts section.

Primary Factors Modified to Increase Peel Depth

• Greater number of layers

Increasing the number of layers, where a layer is defined as complete coverage of the treatment area with chemical peel, deposits a greater quantity of product on the skin and thereby increases the depth of peel penetration. Many other factors also increase the depth of penetration with blended peels and they are outlined in the Factors Influencing the Depth of Chemical Peel Penetration section in Chemical Peel Introduction and Foundation Concepts.

Practical Considerations with Self-Neutralizing Blended Peels

• **Formulations.** Self-neutralizing blended peels commonly contain salicylic acid (SA), TCA, LA, and other acids in relatively low concentrations compared to single acid preparations. They are usually solutions or gels. Examples of self-neutralizing blended peels include TCA 10% with LA 20%, SA 20% with mandelic acid 10%, and retinol 10% with LA 20%. Self-neutralizing blended peels may also contain additional functional ingredients that target specific skin conditions such as melanogenesis inhibitors (e.g., hydroquinone and kojic acid), hydrating agents (e.g., soy isoflavones), anti-inflammatory (e.g., bisabolol) and antioxidant ingredients (e.g., L-ascorbic acid).
• **Patch testing.** Patch testing is recommended for all chemical peels (see Patch Testing, Chemical Peel Introduction and Foundation Concepts section, for testing methodology and interpretation).
• **Toxicity and adverse reactions.** Salicylate toxicity, or salicylism, is extremely rare with blended peels containing salicylic acid due to the relatively low concentration found in blended peels. Signs of salicylism include nausea, disorientation, and tinnitus, and cases have been reported in patients with non-intact skin. Large body surfaces (e.g., more than 25% total body surface area, such as a whole back) are avoided to reduce the risk of toxicity. See Table 2, Chemical Peel Introduction and Foundation Concepts section, for body surface areas.

Practical Considerations with Blended Peels

• **Clinical endpoints with blended peels.** Mild erythema is the desired endpoint for most blended peels. Clinical endpoints are also determined by the constituent ingredients in a peel and the peel's specific formulation. Providers are advised to follow the manufacturer's recommendations for endpoints with the exact formulation being used.
  • Blended peels containing higher strength TCA (such as TCA 15–20%) may have level 1 frosting (faint skin whitening with patchy erythema), but this is uncommon.

- Blended peels containing salicylic acid may form a white powdery precipitate (pseudofrost), but not reliably.
- Blended peels containing retinoids typically leave a temporary yellow discoloration to the skin.
- **Neutralization with blended peels.**
  - Blended peels containing glycolic acid require neutralization and their procedure for use is similar to single ingredient glycolic acid peels (see the Alpha Hydroxy Acid Peel: Glycolic Acid chapter).
  - Blended peels that do not contain glycolic acid do not typically require neutralization and are discussed in this chapter and in the Jessner Peel chapter.

Performing a Superficial Chemical Peel Using a Blended Peel Containing TCA 6% with Lactic Acid 12%

The following procedure uses TCA 6% with lactic acid 12% (Sensi Peel by PCA SKIN) as an example of a self-neutralizing blended chemical peel. Techniques vary for products from different manufacturers, and providers are advised to familiarize themselves with protocols for the specific agent used and to follow manufacturer's instructions.

Preparation: Position, Drape, Cleanse and Degrease Skin, Apply Eye Protection and Petrolatum

1. Setup all products necessary for the procedure within arms' reach.
2. Position the patient supine on the treatment table.
3. Using a headband or surgical cap, secure patient's hair away from the face.
4. Drape a towel across the neck and chest to protect patient's clothing.
5. Apply gentle cleanser to the face with gloved hands and use fingertips to rub the cleanser in small circular motions. Remove using 4×4 non-woven gauze moistened with water.
6. Cleanse the face a second time with an alpha hydroxy cleanser using the method above.
7. Degrease the skin with an astringent toner using 4×4 non-woven gauze. The same application technique that will be used for the peeling solution should also be used to degrease the skin, to reinforce the application method (see step 13 below). Allow the skin to dry.
8. Examine the skin again and limit treatment areas if necessary.
   - Acne lesions may be treated, but it is advisable to avoid treatment of all other areas with non-intact skin.
9. Cover the patient's eyes with disposable adhesive pads or moistened gauze for protection.
10. Apply petrolatum sparingly to areas of potential pooling using a cotton-tipped applicator including the lateral canthal creases, nasolabial folds particularly at the ala, oral commissures, and marionette lines.

Chemical Peel Application

11. Select the appropriate peel and desired applicator. A 4×4 non-woven gauze applicator is used here.
12. Dampen the 4×4 non-woven gauze with the peel by inverting the peel bottle directly onto the gauze approximately 4 to 5 times to form a diamond pattern of solution on the gauze. Dry gloved hands on a towel.

13. Apply the blended peel evenly to the face with the 4 × 4 non-woven. The method of application demonstrated in this chapter is slightly altered from the method outlined in the Chemical Peel Procedure Overview, Chemical Peel Introduction and Foundation Concepts section.
    - **Quadrant 1, forehead.** Using firm even pressure, sweep the gauze from the eyebrow up to hairline.
    - **Quadrant 2, cheek.** Sweep the gauze from the temple to the jawline on one side of the face. The cheek can be covered using horizontal sweeps either from medial to lateral or from superior to inferior.
    - **Quadrant 3, cheek.** Repeat for the contralateral cheek.
    - **Quadrant 4, medial face.** Sweep the gauze down the dorsum of the nose, along each nasal sidewall, above the upper lip, and then across the chin.
    - **Feather the edge of the treatment** area with chemical peel by lightly sweeping the gauze 1 cm below the jawline. This helps avoid a possible line of demarcation between treated and untreated skin, although this is not common when using blended peel solutions.
    - **Open bottles or soaked applicators should never be passed over the patient's eyes.** If peel solution enters the patient's eyes, copiously flush the eye immediately with normal saline solution or water.
    - If deep wrinkles are present, stretch the skin while applying the peel to reduce potential pooling of peel solution to pool in wrinkles.
14. After 1 layer of the peel has been applied to the treatment area, begin the timer to monitor the duration of the procedure.
15. Provide the patient with a handheld fan. Self-fanning reduces discomfort and serves as a distraction.
16. Communicate with the patient regarding any sensations or discomfort they may be feeling using a pain scale of 1 to 10.
    - Mild tingling, itching, burning, or stinging sensations are common and typically peak 2–3 minutes after application, and then subside.
    - Discomfort up to a 5 or 6 out of 10 is acceptable.
17. Observe the skin throughout treatment for desirable and undesirable clinical endpoints.

Desirable clinical endpoints for self-neutralizing blended chemical peels include

- **Mild erythema**
- **White crystal residue ("pseudofrost")**

Note: A pseudofrost with blended peels containing salicylic acid may be visible.

Undesirable clinical endpoints for self-neutralizing blended chemical peels include

- **Blistering/vesiculation** which is indicative of epidermolysis
- **Excessive patient discomfort** with pain greater than 6 out of 10, or overly irritating sensations

18. Wait 2–3 minutes to ensure the peel has fully penetrated. Assess the skin for the degree of erythema. Mild erythema is the typical desired endpoint for blended peels. A white powdery precipitate can be seen with blended peels containing SA, referred to as pseudofrosting. A white discoloration with blended peels containing TCA is also possible, referred to as frosting; however, this is uncommon. A pseudofrost can be wiped off with dry gauze whereas true frosting cannot be wiped off.
19. Acne lesions may frost due to deeper peel penetration.
20. Apply additional peel layers to the face, for a total of 2–3 layers using the above technique. Avoid acne lesions that have already frosted.

Termination

21. The chemical peel procedure is terminated if/when
    - Desired clinical endpoint of mild erythema or a pseudofrost is visible or
    - Undesired endpoints occur including blistering/vesiculation, or excessive patient discomfort
22. Self-neutralizing blended peels do not require application of a neutralizing agent.
23. If undesirable clinical endpoints occur, remove peel product from the skin using dry gauze.
    - In the case of extreme discomfort or concern that a patient is allergic to an ingredient, some providers choose to rinse the skin using gauze saturated with water. Place a stack of dry 4 × 4 gauze into a small bowl and pour water into the bowl. Using the moistened gauze, briskly wipe the face from the center to the periphery. Repeat using freshly saturated gauze 2–3 times or more. Wrapped ice packs or cold moistened towels may be applied to the face if necessary to reduce discomfort. Application of water to a self-neutralizing blended peel can increase the patient's level of discomfort by reactivating the acid, but if done quickly with large amounts of water can dilute the acid and improve patient comfort.
    - The patient may continue fanning until comfortable.
    - Apply soothing topical products as outlined below if undesirable endpoints occur:
      - **Moderate–severe erythema:** apply a high potency steroid cream (e.g., triamcinolone 0.5%), avoiding the periocular area.
      - **Moderate erythema:** apply a medium potency steroid cream (e.g., triamcinolone 0.1%), avoiding the periocular area.
      - **Mild erythema:** apply either a low potency steroid cream (e.g., hydrocortisone 0.5% to 2.5%) or a soothing moisturizer (e.g., SkinCeuticals Epidermal Repair or PCA SKIN's ReBalance or Calming Balm).
24. Daily topical skin care products with active ingredients that are typically intended for home use such as vitamin C antioxidant serums or pigment gels can be applied after the peel application. Follow specific manufacturer guidelines for application of active products immediately following peel application to ensure compatibility with the peel.

Boost (Optional)

25. **Retinoid peels** can be applied after the blended peel, if there are no undesirable endpoints, to increase cell turnover and speed the desquamation process.
    - It is advisable to first perform the blended peel procedure without a retinoid booster to ensure tolerability to the primary peel.
    - Dry the skin by fanning prior to applying the retinoid booster peel. See Retinoid Peel chapter for information on applying booster peels.

- Providers are encouraged to follow manufacturer instructions for using a booster retinoid peel with the primary peel to confirm the appropriateness of combining the peels and ensure compatibility.

Topical Product Application

26. **Soothe.** Assess the skin for the degree of erythema and apply a soothing topical product as outlined below:
    - **Moderate–severe erythema:** apply a high potency steroid cream (e.g., triamcinolone 0.5%), avoiding the periocular area.
    - **Moderate erythema:** apply a medium potency steroid cream (e.g., triamcinolone 0.1%), avoiding the periocular area.
    - **Mild erythema:** apply either a low potency steroid cream (hydrocortisone 0.5% to 2.5%) or a soothing non-occlusive moisturizer (e.g., SkinCeuticals Epidermal Repair or PCA SKIN's Calming Balm).
27. **Protect.** Apply a **broad-spectrum sunscreen** of SPF 30 or higher containing zinc oxide or titanium dioxide at the conclusion of treatment (e.g., products by Skin Medica, Solar Protection, SkinCeuticals or PCA SKIN) to protect the skin from UV exposure.

Aftercare

- Patients requiring topical steroids immediately after treatment will benefit from inclusion of a topical steroid in their postprocedure home care regimen to further reduce erythema and hence the risk of postinflammatory hyperpigmentation.
- Acne lesions that have frosted may form a crust 1–2 days after treatment. This is managed with daily application of bacitracin until resolved.

See Aftercare, Chemical Peel Introduction and Foundation Concepts section for aftercare instructions.

Treatment Intervals, and Complications and Management

See Chemical Peel Introduction and Foundation Concepts for these sections.

Progressive Peeling: Increasing Intensity of Subsequent Treatments

Self-neutralizing blended peel treatments can be intensified at subsequent visits by increasing the depth of peel penetration in several possible ways:

- **Number of layers.** Applying more layers is usually the first step in increasing treatment intensity with self-neutralizing blended peels. For example, if a treatment is terminated after 1–2 layers with TCA 6% with lactic acid 12%, the goal for the subsequent treatment may be 4 layers with the same peel.
- **Peel concentration.** Treatment intensity may be increased by using a blended peel with higher percentages of similar ingredients on subsequent visits. For example, if a patient tolerates TCA 6% with lactic acid 12% with 4 layers (e.g., PCA SKIN's Sensi Peel), on the next visit the TCA 10% with lactic acid 20% (e.g., PCA SKIN's Ultra Peel I) could be used.

- **Boost.** An additional retinoid peel may be applied after the final layer of a TCA 6% with lactic acid 12% blended peel to increase treatment intensity and enhance desquamation. For example, after a treatment with 4 layers of a TCA 6% with lactic acid 12% blended peel, the subsequent treatment may be intensified by applying a non-prescription retinoid such as retinol 10% at the booster step of the peel process. At the next visit, the treatment may be further intensified by applying retinol 10% with lactic acid 20% (e.g., PCA SKIN's Esthetique Peel). If the prior treatment is tolerated, a prescription-strength retinoic acid 0.3% may be used as the booster peel at a subsequent visit (for Fitzpatrick skin types I–III).
- **Microdermabrasion pretreatment.** Microdermabrasion can be used as part of skin preparation prior to the application of a blended peel to allow for more even acid penetration and increase the depth of penetration. For example, two passes with a microdermabrasion using a mild–moderate abrasive element with mild–moderate vacuum setting may be performed immediately prior to a blended peel to intensify the treatment. Use of established manufacturer protocols is recommended when combining these two exfoliation modalities as peel characteristics and depth of penetration can be significantly altered by the lack of the stratum corneum.
- **Modify one treatment parameter at a time** (e.g., number of layers, boost, or pretreatment exfoliation) to increase treatment intensity in as safe and controlled manner as possible. Once the desired number of layers is reached, the intensity of the subsequent treatment can be increased either with pretreatment exfoliation (microdermabrasion) or by using a booster peel.
- **Treatment intensity** may be increased at a subsequent visit only if a patient has demonstrated tolerability to a given peel procedure. Skin is dynamic and variables outside of the providers control may also change, such as patients' preprocedure product regimen, all of which can alter the skin and its response to chemical peel treatments. Therefore, it may not be possible to increase treatment intensity at every visit.

Financial Considerations and Coding

Charges for blended peels vary by geographic region and typically range from $95 to $200 per treatment. Chemical peels are often performed and charged as a series of six treatments to help achieve the best possible results and ensure high patient and provider satisfaction.

Supply Sources

See Appendix 8, Chemical Peel and Topical Product Supply Sources.

Chapter 7

Retinoid Peel: Retinol

Chemical Peel	Neutralization Required	Endpoint Desired	Skin Whitening Desired	Discomfort	Desquamation
Retinoids (retinoic acid and retinol)	No	Mild erythema and yellow tint	No	+	Yes

+ Mild, ++ Moderate, +++ Intense.

Retinoid peeling agents are usually comprised of retinoic acid, retinol, or blends of retinoids (such as retinol retinyl acetate and retinyl palmitate). Retinoid peels can be used alone, but more often are used as a "booster" and layered over other superficial peels, such as alpha hydroxy acids, beta hydroxy acids, Jessner's peel, and blended peels, to intensify treatments and enhance desquamation. Booster peels are not typically performed after higher strength TCA 20% peels.

Chemical Peel Selection, Contraindications, Equipment, Preprocedure Checklist, Preprocedure Skin Care Products, Patch Testing, Steps for Performing a Chemical Peel Procedure, Overview of Chemical Peel Procedure

See Chemical Peel Introduction and Foundation Concepts section.

Primary Factors Modified to Increase Peel Depth

- Chemical peel concentration
- Duration of application

Many other factors can increase retinoid peel depth and they are outlined in the Factors Influencing the Depth of Chemical Peel Penetration in the Chemical Peel Introduction and Foundation Concepts section.

Other Practical Considerations with Retinoid Peels

- **Formulations.** Retinoid peels range from solutions to creams. Retinol is one of the most common non-prescription retinoid peels, typically used in concentrations of 10–15%. Prescription strength retinoid peels are available, such as retinoic acid 0.3%, as well as blended retinoid peels, such as retinol 10% and lactic acid 20%. Application techniques vary according to the consistency of the product. Solutions may be applied using the technique for peel application described in other chapters, such as the Beta Hydroxy Acid chapter. The technique for application of a cream retinoid is outlined in this chapter.
- **Patch testing.** Patch testing is recommended for all chemical peels (see Patch Testing, Chemical Peel Introduction and Foundation Concepts section, for testing methodology and interpretation).

Performing a Booster Chemical Peel Using Retinol 10%

The following procedure uses retinol 10% cream (by PCA SKIN) as an example of a retinoid chemical peel booster, to be applied after a primary superficial peel. Providers are encouraged to follow manufacturer's instructions for using a booster retinoid peel with the primary peel to confirm the appropriateness of combining the peels and to ensure compatibility.

Primary Peel Preparation, Application, and Termination

1. Complete the primary peel procedure with neutralization if indicated.
2. Ensure the skin is dry.
3. Examine the skin in the treatment area once again and limit treatment areas if necessary.
4. If there are no undesirable endpoints, proceed with booster retinoid peel.

Boost

5. Select the appropriate retinoid peel; a retinol 10% cream is used here.
6. Creams are most easily applied using gloved hands. Dispense a nickel-sized amount of retinol cream onto a gloved hand. Place an equal sized amount in each of the four quadrants (see below) and disperse using fingertips in small circular motions:
   - **Quadrant 1, forehead.**
   - **Quadrant 2, cheek.**
   - **Quadrant 3, cheek.** Repeat for the contralateral cheek.
   - **Quadrant 4, medial face.** First apply down the dorsum of the nose, along each nasal sidewall, above the upper lip, and then across the chin.
   - Place a small amount along the jaw line to feather the edges of the treatment area.
   - **Open bottles or soaked applicators should never be passed over the patient's eyes.** If peel solution enters the patient's eyes, copiously flush the eye immediately with normal saline solution or water.
7. Fanning is rarely required, as retinol peels are associated with minimal discomfort.
8. Communicate with the patient regarding any sensations or discomfort they may be feeling using a pain scale of 1 to 10.
   - Minimal tingling or warming sensations may be reported, which usually subsides within 1–2 minutes.
   - Discomfort up to a 3 or 4 out of 10 is acceptable.

9. Observe the skin throughout treatment for desirable and undesirable clinical endpoints.

> **Desirable** clinical endpoints for retinoid chemical peels include
>
> - **Mild erythema**
> - **Slight yellow coloration**
>
> **Undesirable** clinical endpoints for retinoid chemical peels include
>
> - **Blistering/vesiculation,** which is indicative of epidermolysis
> - **Excessive patient discomfort** with pain greater than 5 out of 10, or overly irritating sensations

10. A temporary yellow discoloration of the skin is immediately visible due to the yellow color of retinoid peels.
11. Cream-based retinoid boosters are applied in one single layer.
12. The skin will feel slightly tacky once the peel has dried.

Termination

13. The chemical peel procedure is terminated if/when
    - Undesired endpoints occur including blistering/vesiculation, whitening of the skin, or excessive patient discomfort.
14. Retinoid peels are self-neutralizing and therefore do not require application of a neutralizing agent.
15. If undesirable clinical endpoints occur, remove peel product from the skin using dry gauze. Then rinse the skin using gauze saturated with water. Place a stack of dry 4 × 4 gauze into a small bowl and pour water into the bowl. Using the moistened gauze, briskly wipe the face from the center to the periphery. Repeat using freshly saturated gauze 2–3 times or more. Wrapped ice packs or cold moistened towels may be applied to the face if necessary to reduce discomfort. Fanning may be continued as desired for comfort.

Topical Product Application

16. **Soothe.** Assess the skin for the degree of erythema and apply a soothing topical product as outlined below:
    - **Moderate–severe erythema:** apply a high potency steroid cream (e.g., triamcinolone 0.5%), avoiding the periocular area.
    - **Moderate erythema:** apply a medium potency steroid cream (e.g., triamcinolone 0.1%), avoiding the periocular area.
    - **Mild erythema:** apply either a low potency steroid cream (e.g., hydrocortisone 0.5% to 2.5%) or a soothing moisturizer (e.g., SkinCeuticals Epidermal Repair or PCA SKIN's Calming Balm).
17. **Protect.** Apply a **broad-spectrum sunscreen** of SPF 30 or higher containing zinc oxide or titanium dioxide at the conclusion of treatment (e.g., products by Skin Medica, Solar Protection, SkinCeuticals or PCA SKIN) to protect the skin from UV exposure.

Aftercare, Treatment Intervals, and Complications

- Instruct the patient to remove the peel at home by cleansing their face 4–8 hours after application, depending on manufacturer recommendations.

See Aftercare, Chemical Peel Introduction and Foundation Concepts section for aftercare instructions and the other sections listed.

Progressive Peeling: Increasing Intensity of Subsequent Treatments

The intensity of a retinoid booster peel treatment can be increased in several possible ways at subsequent visits, by increasing

- **Peel concentration.** Treatment intensity is usually increased by using a stronger retinoid. For example, after a treatment with a primary blended peel of TCA 10% and lactic acid 6%, the subsequent treatment may be intensified by applying a non-prescription retinoid such as retinol 10% at the booster step of the peel process. At the next visit, the treatment may be further intensified by applying retinol 15% with lactic acid 10%. If the prior treatment is tolerated, prescription-strength retinoic acid 0.3% may be used as the booster at the subsequent visit (for Fitzpatrick skin types I–III).
- **Duration of application.** The treatment intensity can be increased by instructing the patient to leave the retinoid peel on for a longer duration. For example, after a treatment with a primary SA 30% peel and retinol 10% left on for 4 hours, the subsequent treatment may be intensified by leaving the peel on for 8 hours.
- **Modify one treatment parameter at a time** (e.g., concentration or duration of application) to increase treatment intensity in as safe and controlled manner as possible.
- **Treatment intensity** may be increased at a subsequent visit only if a patient has demonstrated tolerability to a given peel procedure. Skin is dynamic and variables outside of the providers control may also change, such as patients' preprocedure product regimen, all of which can alter the skin and its response to chemical peel treatments. Therefore, it may not be possible to increase treatment intensity at every visit.

Financial Considerations and Coding

Charges for retinoid peels vary by geographic region and typically range from $65 to $150 per treatment when performed alone, and when used as a booster $45 to $55. Chemical peels are often performed and charged as a series of six treatments to help achieve the best possible results and ensure high patient and provider satisfaction.

Supply Sources

See Appendix 8, Chemical Peel and Topical Product Supply Sources.

Microdermabrasion

Microdermabrasion (MDA) is a mechanical exfoliation procedure for superficial skin resurfacing which utilizes a refined abrasive element, such as a diamond-tipped pad or aerosolized crystals, to gently remove the outermost skin layers. This controlled wounding process stimulates cell renewal with regeneration of a healthier epidermis and dermis. Microdermabrasion is used for treatment of photoaging, hyperpigmentation, and acne, as well as fine lines and superficial scars. It is one of the most commonly performed aesthetic procedures in the United States with nearly half a million treatments performed annually, according to data from the American Society for Aesthetic Plastic Surgery. This practical guide focuses on treatment of photodamaged skin and utilizes an integrated approach, combining MDA with chemical peels and topical home care products to maximize results.

Patient Selection

While almost any patient will derive benefit from microdermabrasion, patients with mild to moderate photoaging changes such as solar lentigines, dullness, and rough skin texture (e.g., Glogau types I and II), as well as acneic conditions, typically derive the most noticeable benefits (see Introduction Concepts and Foundation Concepts for a description of Glogau types). Results are cumulative and a series of treatments are necessary for noticeable improvements. Microdermabrasion can also improve fine lines, enlarged pores and atrophic scars; however, results are not comparable to those achieved with deeper skin resurfacing procedures such as medium depth peels or laser resurfacing. Discussion of expectations at the time of consultation and commitment to a series of treatments is essential to ensure success with microdermabrasion.

Patients of all Fitzpatrick skin types (I–VI) may be treated with MDA (see Introduction and Foundation Concepts for a description of Fitzpatrick skin types). However, it is advisable to treat darker skin types (IV–VI) conservatively to minimize the risks of pigmentary changes such as postinflammatory hyperpigmentation (PIH). Treating patients with erythematous conditions such as rosacea, telangiectasia, and Poikiloderma of Civatte with MDA is controversial. Clearly, overly aggressive treatments can accentuate erythema. However, patients with erythema have impaired barrier function and mild MDA treatments strengthening the epidermal barrier may ultimately reduce skin sensitivity and erythema. Some providers, therefore, do perform MDA on patients with erythematous conditions using conservative settings in areas of high vascularity such as the midface and chin, and higher settings around the periphery of the face. Mild treatments are also recommended when treating elderly patients with thin skin to reduce the risk of abrasions.

Indications

- Photodamage
- Rough texture

111

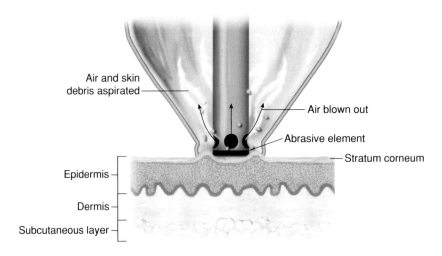

Air and skin debris aspirated

Air blown out

Abrasive element

Stratum corneum

Epidermis

Dermis

Subcutaneous layer

FIGURE 1 ● Microdermabrasion exfoliation process.

- Fine lines
- Hyperpigmentation
- Dull, sallow skin color
- Enlarged pores
- Acne simplex
- Acne vulgaris (not pustules)
- Superficial acne scars
- Keratosis pilaris
- Thickened scaling skin (e.g., ichthyosis)
- Dry skin (xerosis)
- Seborrheic keratosis scaling
- Enhanced penetration of topical products and chemical peels

Mechanism of Action

Most MDA devices have a closed-loop vacuum system that draws the skin against an abrasive element at the handpiece tip. As the handpiece is moved across the skin, the outermost layers are removed and the cellular debris is aspirated into a container that is disposed of after treatment (Fig. 1). Common abrasive elements used in MDA devices include diamond-tipped pads, crystal pads, aerosolized crystals, and bristles.

Depth of Penetration

Skin resurfacing with MDA ranges from removal of the stratum corneum (very superficial resurfacing) to removal of the entire epidermis (superficial resurfacing). Standardized definitions for resurfacing depths are illustrated in the Anatomy section, Figure 4. Greater depth of penetration into the skin offers more significant improvements. While there are few risks with MDA, greater depth of penetration is associated with greater risks of complications.

Each pass of a medical-grade MDA handpiece removes approximately 15 μm of skin. Two passes typically exfoliate the stratum corneum, and four passes exfoliate the whole epidermis. For example, the SilkPeel MDA fully exfoliates the stratum corneum after two passes at a vacuum setting of 5 psi (260 mm Hg) using a 60-grit treatment head.

Several factors increase the depth of penetration with MDA devices including:

- Higher vacuum pressures
- Greater number of passes, where a pass is defined as contiguous coverage of a treatment area
- Treatment head abrasiveness
- Greater downward pressure on the skin (for devices with non-recessed tips)

Microdermabrasion Devices

The first MDA devices used aerosolized crystal particles (e.g., aluminum oxide) as the abrasive element which were blown across the skin and aspirated. While these devices are still in use, particle-free MDA devices have become widely adopted as they pose no risks of dust inhalation or corneal abrasion, which are associated with aerosolized crystal particles.

Particle-free MDA devices utilize diamond- or crystal-covered pads, or bristles in their treatment heads. Figure 2 shows an MDA handpiece (SilkPeel) and treatment heads with diamond-covered pads that range in coarseness from smooth (no diamond chips), fine (120 grit), to coarse (30 grit). Treatment heads for most devices are reusable and can be sterilized after the procedure. Devices utilizing ultrasonic mechanical oscillation have also been introduced as a means of exfoliation, but there are few studies on their efficacy.

Some MDA devices simultaneously exfoliate and apply topical products to the skin (specifically referred to as "Dermalinfusion" by Envy Medical). These systems take advantage of the disruption to the epidermal barrier that occurs with removal of the stratum corneum to enhance delivery of topical products to the skin. If using a MDA

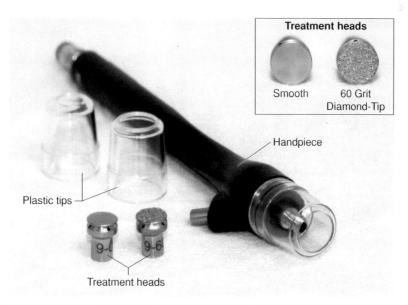

FIGURE 2 ● Microdermabrasion handpiece and diamond-tipped treatment heads. (SilkPeel by Envy Medical, Courtesy of Rebecca Small, MD)

device that does not dispense solutions, topical corrective products may be applied after completion of the MDA treatment. Products are selected based on the presenting signs and may enhance results for conditions such as dehydration, hyperpigmentation, and acne.

MDA devices are classified as type I devices by the U.S. Food and Drug Administration (FDA), which do not require the manufacturer to establish performance standards or perform clinical trials to demonstrate efficacy. Most MDA machines are manufactured for aestheticians with a few medical-grade devices manufactured for physicians. Medical-grade MDA devices are capable of deeper exfoliation due to higher vacuum pressures and more abrasive treatment heads (see Appendix 7, Microdermabrasion Supply Sources, for a list of MDA device manufacturers).

Alternative Therapies

Superficial chemical peels provide a similar depth of skin resurfacing as microdermabrasion. Dermaplaning is another superficial resurfacing procedure with a similar depth of resurfacing, which uses a specialized scalpel blade that is gently scraped across the skin. It is useful for patients with erythematous conditions such as rosacea.

More aggressive skin resurfacing procedures such as medium-depth chemical peels, dermabrasion, and laser resurfacing offer significantly greater reduction of wrinkles and improvements in photodamaged skin, but require longer recovery times and have increased risks of complications.

Advantages of Microdermabrasion

- Controlled depth of exfoliation
- Safe for all Fitzpatrick skin types (I–VI)
- Minimal to no discomfort during the procedure
- No anesthesia required
- Minimal risk of complications
- No recovery time postprocedure (e.g., for skin flaking and peeling as with chemical peels)
- May be combined with other aesthetic treatments, particularly topical products and chemical peels, for enhanced results
- Procedural proficiency rapidly acquired

Disadvantages of Microdermabrasion

- MDA devices are relatively costly (compared to chemical peels)
- Additional costs for disposable supplies such as topical solutions
- Results are subtle and cumulative, requiring a series of treatments for noticeable improvements

Contraindications

- Pregnancy or nursing
- Active infection (e.g., herpes simplex, impetigo or cellulitis) or open wound in the treatment area
- Keloidal or hypertrophic scarring
- Melanoma (or lesions suspected for melanoma), basal cell, or squamous cell carcinoma in the treatment area

- Dermatoses (e.g., vitiligo, active psoriasis, or atopic dermatitis) in the treatment area
- Impaired healing (e.g., due to immunosuppression)
- Skin atrophy (e.g., chronic steroid use or genetic syndromes such as Ehlers–Danlos)
- Bleeding abnormality (e.g., thrombocytopenia or anticoagulant use)
- Uncontrolled systemic condition
- Deep chemical peel, dermabrasion, or radiation therapy in the treatment area within the preceding 6 months
- Isotretinoin (Accutane) use within the past 6 months
- Severe pustular acne
- Excessive laxity and skin folds
- Insufficient sun protection
- Unrealistic expectations
- Body dysmorphic disorder

Equipment

- MDA device with abrasive element
- Headband
- Facial wash and astringent toner to cleanse and degrease the treatment area
- Towel to drape the patient
- Non-sterile gloves
- Eye protection for the patient (adhesive eye pads, goggles, or moist gauze)
- 4 × 4 gauze
- Broad-spectrum sunscreen of SPF 30 or greater containing zinc oxide or titanium dioxide (e.g., products by Solar Protection, SkinCeuticals and PCA SKIN) and a nonocclusive soothing moisturizer (e.g., SkinCeutical's Epidermal Repair or PCA SKIN's ReBalance) for postprocedure application
- Saline eye wash

Preprocedure Checklist

- Review the patient's medical and cosmetic history (an example of a Patient Intake Form is provided in Appendix 2).
- Perform an aesthetic consultation (see Introduction and Foundation Concepts, Consultation section).
- Determine the patient's Fitzpatrick skin type and Glogau score (see Introduction and Foundation Concepts, Consultation section).
- Examine the treatment areas and assess for the presence of wrinkles, acne, scars, benign vascular or pigmented lesions, oiliness/dryness, and other skin conditions. An example of a Skin Analysis Form is provided in Appendix 3.
- Obtain informed consent (see Introduction and Foundation Concepts). An example of a Consent for Skin Care Treatments is provided in Appendix 4.
- Pretreatment photographs are recommended (see Introduction and Foundation Concepts).
- A broad-spectrum sunscreen of SPF 30 or greater containing zinc oxide or titanium dioxide is used daily prior to and for the duration of treatments.
- Two weeks prior to the procedure, patients are advised to discontinue tanning and direct sun exposure, and avoid for the duration of treatments.

- One to two weeks prior to treatment, patients are advised to discontinue products containing high strength alpha hydroxy acids (such as glycolic and lactic acids) and prescription retinoids (such as Retin-A, Renova, and Differin).
- Two days prior to the procedure, a prophylactic antiviral medication (e.g., acyclovir 400 mg or valacyclovir 500 mg, 1 tablet 2 times per day) is begun for patients with a history of herpes simplex or varicella in or around the treatment area, and continued for 3 days postprocedure.
- On the day of the procedure, patients are advised to wash the treatment area, and remove facial jewelry and contact lenses.

Overview of Microdermabrasion Procedure

- The area within which MDA treatments can be safely performed on the face is referred to as the microdermabrasion Safety Zone (Fig. 3). All regions of the face may be treated apart from the area within the bony orbital rim and, for most devices, the lips. MDA devices that have non-abrasive smooth treatment heads may be used on the lips (Fig. 2). MDA may be performed on the face, neck, chest, hands, back, and almost any area of the body requiring exfoliation.
- Anesthesia is not necessary with MDA treatments.
- Treatment intensity ranges from mild to aggressive and is selected based on the presenting skin condition and treatment area, as outlined below:

Treatment Intensity	MDA Settings	Skin Conditions Treated
Mild	2 passes, mild abrasive element, low vacuum	Papular acne, erythema, darker Fitzpatrick skin types (IV–VI), thin skin
Moderate	2–4 passes, moderate abrasive element, moderate vacuum	Hyperpigmentation, rough skin, fine lines, coarse pores, comedonal acne, keratosis pilaris, combination treatments when MDA is followed by a chemical peel or for photodynamic therapy
Aggressive	4 or more passes, coarse abrasive element, high vacuum	Superficial acne scars (face) and non-facial hyperkeratotic areas such as elbows, knees, and pedal calluses

Performing the Microdermabrasion Procedure

The following recommendations are guidelines for MDA treatments on the face using a particle-free, diamond-tipped device, which simultaneously applies topical solutions (SilkPeel by Envy Medical). Recommended treatment parameters vary according to the device used, and manufacturer guidelines for the SilkPeel or other device used should be followed at the time of treatment.

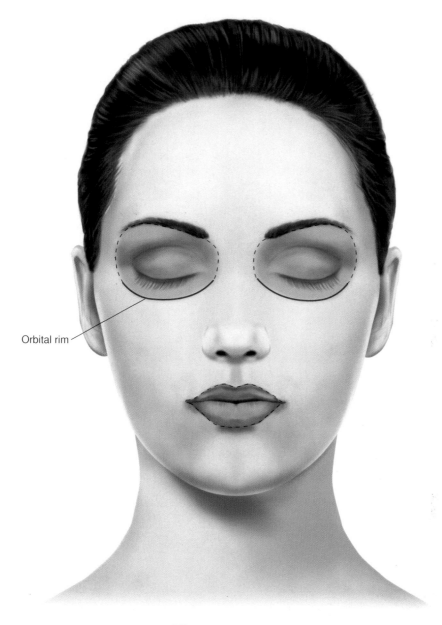

Orbital rim

= Non-treatment areas

FIGURE 3 ● Microdermabrasion Safety Zone.

1. Position the patient supine on the treatment table.
2. Use a headband to pull hair away from the patient's face.
3. Cover the patient's eyes with protective eyewear such as adhesive eye pads or moist gauze.
4. Cleanse the treatment area with a gentle cleanser, then degrease with alcohol or an astringent toner. Wait for the skin to dry completely before starting the procedure.
5. Select the treatment head size based on the treatment area.
   - With the SilkPeel, the 6 mm head is typically used for face, neck, chest, and hands, and the larger 9 mm head is used for other body areas.

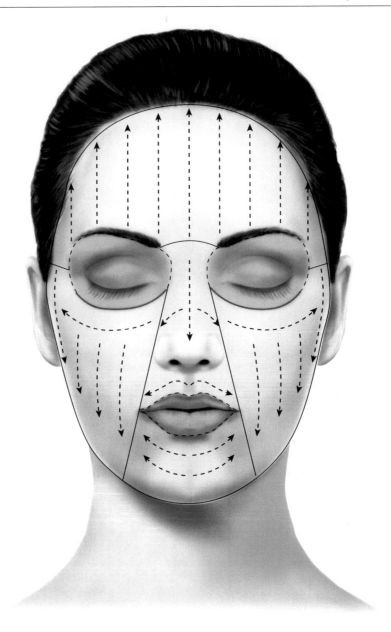

⬚ = Non-treatment areas   – – → = Microdermabrasion handpiece direction

FIGURE 4 ● Directional guide for microdermabrasion.

6. Select the treatment head coarseness based on the desired treatment intensity. Suggestions for treatment parameters using the SilkPeel MDA are shown below.

Treatment Intensity	Treatment Head Coarseness	Vacuum Pressure (psi)
Mild	140 grit	3.0–3.5
Moderate	120 grit	3.5–4.0
Aggressive	60–100 grit	4.0–5.0

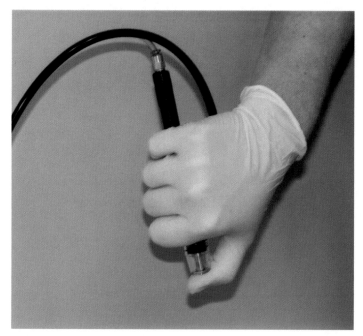

FIGURE 5 ● Handpiece occlusion for selection of microdermabrasion vacuum settings. (SilkPeel by Envy Medical, Courtesy of Rebecca Small, MD)

7. Set the vacuum pressure by inverting the handpiece and occluding the tip with a gloved finger (Fig. 5). The strength of the vacuum affects the depth of resurfacing, and small adjustments in this parameter can fine-tune the intensity of a treatment. Conservative vacuum settings are recommended for initial treatments. Consider decreasing vacuum settings when treating thin-skinned areas such as the periorbital area.

8. Select a topical product appropriate for the presenting condition and then select a flow rate of infusion per the manufacturer's guidelines.
   - **Hyperpigmentation** may be treated with lightening agents such as hydroquinone, kojic acid, arbutin, or brightening peptides (e.g., decapeptide-12).
   - **Dehydration and fine lines** may be treated with hyaluronic acid, allantoin, and glycerin.
   - **Photodamage** may be treated with vitamin C.
   - **Acne** may be treated with erythromycin and salicylic acid.

9. Cover the entire face with contiguous sweeps of the handpiece as shown in Figure 4. Begin at the forehead, then proceed down the nose, cheeks, and lastly around the mouth and chin.

10. Move the handpiece across the skin as follows: stretch the skin between two fingers, and holding the handpiece perpendicular to the skin, bring the tip gently in contact with the skin. Slowly and smoothly move the handpiece across the face using even pressure, parallel to the tension lines between the fingers (Fig. 6). The tip must move across the skin for exfoliation to occur with devices that utilize abrasive pads such as the SilkPeel.

11. Communicate with the patient regarding any discomfort they may be feeling using a pain scale of 1 to 10. Patients typically report minimal to no discomfort.
    - Discomfort up to 4 out of 10 is acceptable.

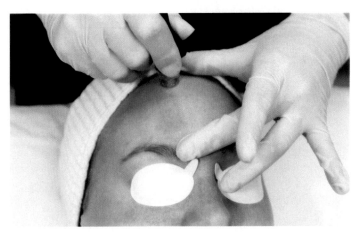

FIGURE 6 ● Technique for microdermabrasion first pass on the face. (Courtesy of Rebecca Small, MD)

12. Observe the skin throughout treatment for desirable and undesirable clinical endpoints.

> **Desirable** clinical endpoints for microdermabrasion include
>
> - **Mild erythema**
>
> **Undesirable** clinical endpoints for microdermabrasion include
>
> - **Petechiae or purpura** (visible as small red dots or bruising, respectively)
> - **Excessive patient discomfort** with pain greater than 5 out of 10, or overly irritating sensations

13. Undesired endpoints indicate overly aggressive treatment. If undesired endpoints occur, reduce treatment intensity by decreasing vacuum pressure and/or grit coarseness and avoid the affected area for the remainder of treatment.
14. After completing treatment of the entire area, perform a second pass to the same treatment area (if undesired endpoints have not occurred) by moving the handpiece perpendicular to the previous handpiece direction (Fig. 7).
15. After the treatment, apply a soothing nonocclusive moisturizer followed by a broad-spectrum sunscreen with SPF 30 or higher containing zinc oxide or titanium dioxide.
16. Sanitize (e.g., using a quaternary ammonium solution, commonly referred to as quats) or sterilize (e.g., by autoclave) reusable equipment parts between treatments per the manufacturer guidelines.

Aftercare

Patients commonly experience mild erythema and/or dryness for up to 3 days after treatment. A broad-spectrum sunscreen with SPF 30 or greater that contains zinc oxide or titanium dioxide (e.g., products by Solar Protection, SkinCeuticals, and PCA SKIN) is recommended daily and throughout the series of treatments. A nonocclusive moisturizer (e.g., SkinCeutical's Epidermal Repair or PCA SKIN's ReBalance) may be applied

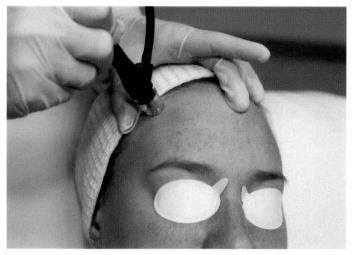

FIGURE 7 ● Technique for microdermabrasion second pass on the face. (Courtesy of Rebecca Small, MD)

in the evening as often as needed for dryness (see Pre and Postprocedure Skin Care Products, in the Skin Care Products section for additional information on postprocedure products). Patients are advised to avoid irritating products such as retinoids, astringent toners, depilatories, and exfoliants such as glycolic acid, for 1–2 weeks. Patients are also advised to avoid direct sun exposure for 4 weeks and for the duration of their treatments. An example of a postprocedure patient handout is provided in Appendix 5, Before and After Instructions for Skin Care Treatments.

Results

Microdermabrasion results are progressive. While improvement in skin texture and skin brightness may be observed after a single treatment, more marked improvements including reduction of hyperpigmentation, acne, and fine lines typically require a series of six treatments.

Figure 8 shows a patient with moderate photodamage with solar lentigines, dullness, and fine lines before (A) and after (B) a series of six treatments using a bristle MDA (DermaSweep) with application of topical solutions during treatment containing hydroxy acids (glycolic, salicylic, and lactic acids) and lightening agents (kojic and azelaic acids, bearberry, and licorice).

Figure 9 shows a patient with acne vulgaris before (A) and after (B) a series of six MDA treatments using a diamond-tipped MDA (SilkPeel) with application of topical solutions during treatment containing hydroxy acids (salicylic and glycolic acids) and lightening agents (kojic acid and arbutin).

Figure 10 shows a patient with a dark Fitzpatrick skin type (V) with solar lentigines and dullness before (A) and after (B) a series of six MDA treatments using a diamond-tipped MDA (SilkPeel) with application of topical solutions during treatment containing a lightening peptide (decapeptide-12).

Increasing Intensity of Subsequent Treatments

At subsequent visits, treatments may be intensified by increasing the number of passes or the treatment head grit coarseness. It is advisable to change only one of these variables at any one time to safely escalate treatment intensity. The skin is

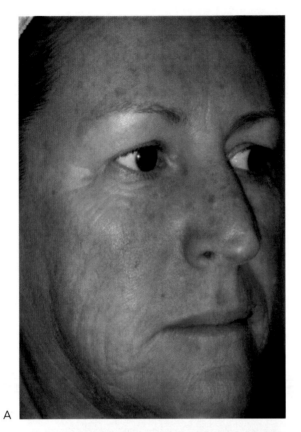

A

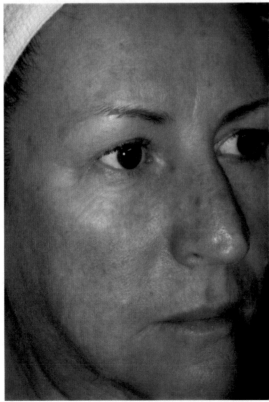

B

FIGURE 8 ● Photodamaged skin with solar lentigines, dullness, and fine lines before **(A)** and after **(B)** six bristle microdermabrasion (DermaSweep) treatments. (Courtesy of DermaSweep)

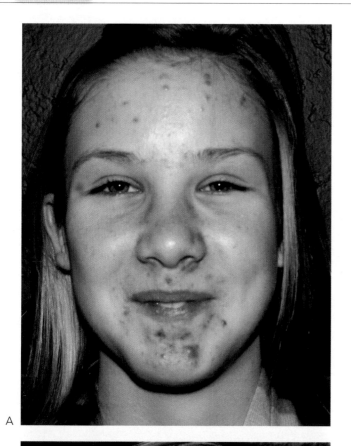

A

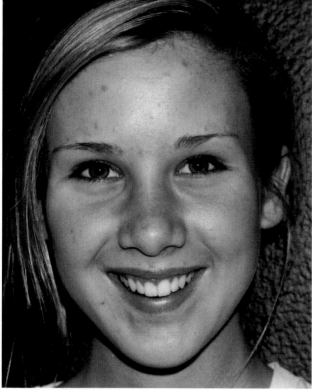

B

FIGURE 9 ● Acne vulgaris before **(A)** and after **(B)** six diamond-tipped microdermabrasion (SilkPeel) treatments. (Courtesy of Envy Medical)

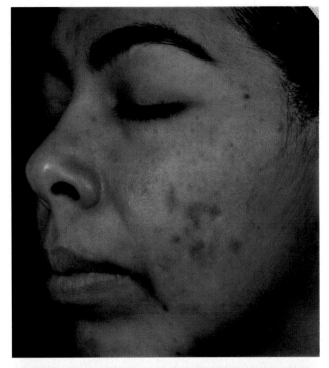

A

B

FIGURE 10 ● Postinflammatory hyperpigmentation and acne in a patient with a dark Fitzpatrick skin type before **(A)** and after **(B)** six diamond-tipped microdermabrasion (SilkPeel) treatments. (Courtesy of A. Bhatia, MD and Envy Medical)

reassessed at each visit prior to treatment, as the condition of skin is dynamic and may vary between treatments, and it may not be possible to increase intensity at each subsequent treatment.

Treatment Intervals

Microdermabrasion treatments may be performed every 2–4 weeks during a treatment series. To maintain results after the initial series treatments may be performed every 4–6 weeks.

Learning the Techniques

Providers are encouraged to practice on the dorsum of the hand to get a feel for moving the tip across the skin with different vacuum pressures. Treating staff and friends initially can aid providers in developing a systematic approach for treating the face and acquiring proficiency with microdermabrasion.

Non-facial Treatment Areas

MDA may be performed on the neck, anterior chest (also called décolletage), hands, back, and almost any area of the body requiring exfoliation. The skin on the body is different from that of the face as it has fewer pilosebaceous units, which are the sites of re-epithelialization and sebum production. Non-facial skin has delayed healing relative to the face, shows less dramatic improvements after treatment, and is more prone to complications such as scarring with overly aggressive treatments. Therefore, it is advisable to treat non-facial areas conservatively.

Neck: position the patient with the chin lifted and extended. Perform 1–2 passes using handpiece sweeps from the chin toward the clavicle.

Chest: perform the first pass with handpiece sweeps from the midline of the chest to the periphery. The second pass sweeps are vertical from the chest to the clavicle.

Hands: position the hand into a fist. Perform 1–2 passes with handpiece sweeps parallel to the forearm.

Advanced Microdermabrasion

As skill and experience are gained with microdermabrasion, providers may choose to combine MDA with other procedures. For example, MDA may be used prior to the application of chemical peels to allow for more even peel application and to enhance the depth of penetration into the skin. It is advisable to use established manufacturer protocols when combining these two exfoliation procedures, as removal of the stratum corneum barrier by MDA can significantly alter the characteristics of a peel.

MDA may also be used as part of photodynamic therapy (PDT). This is an FDA-approved treatment for non-hyperkeratotic actinic keratoses on the face, and PDT is used off-label to enhance light-based photorejuvenation treatments. PDT utilizes application of topical photosensitizing medications such as 5-aminolevulanic acid (Levulan) followed by activation with an appropriate light source such as an intense-pulsed light (IPL), light-emitting diode (LED) or laser. MDA can be performed prior to application of the photosensitizer to enhance product penetration and increase PDT treatment intensity.

Complications and Management

- Pain
- Prolonged erythema
- Postinflammatory hyperpigmentation
- Severe dryness and/or pruritis
- Superficial abrasion
- Infections (e.g., activation of herpes simplex, impetigo, and candidiasis)
- Contact dermatitis
- Urticaria
- Petechiae or purpura
- Remote possibility of scarring or hypopigmentation

Microdermabrasion is a very safe, well-tolerated procedure that has minimal risks of complications. One study of more than 100 patients receiving MDA over a 2-year period reported no instances of infection, long-term hyperpigmentation, or scarring. However, complications are possible with any procedure, and knowledge of these is important to minimize risks and helps ensure the best possible results.

Erythema is anticipated immediately after treatment. The duration of erythema depends on the aggressiveness of the procedure and the reactivity of patients' skin. Most erythema resolves spontaneously within a day, but occasionally may last up to 5 days. If erythema is significant immediately after treatment, ice may be applied to the skin for 15 minutes every hour followed by a topical steroid cream. In the office, a high-potency topical steroid cream may be used (e.g., triamcinolone 0.5%), and the patient may be sent home with a low-potency steroid (e.g., hydrocortisone 2.5% or 1%) to be used twice daily for 3–5 days or until erythema resolves. Prolonged erythema, particularly in patients with darker Fitzpatrick skin types (IV–VI), can lead to PIH. Sun avoidance and use of sunscreen is very important to reduce the risk of PIH when erythema is present.

Hyperpigmentation can be treated with lightening agents such as hydroquinone or cosmeceutical agents such as kojic acid, arbutin, and licorice (see Topical Skin Care Products section for additional information on treatment of hyperpigmentation). Resolution of hyperpigmentation is slower in darker Fitzpatrick skin types (IV–VI) and can take up to several months. In rare instances, hyperpigmentation may be permanent.

Severe dryness and pruritis can be managed with application of moisturizers. Use of occlusive moisturizers, such as Aquaphor, will reduce dryness, but can be associated with acne and milia. Therefore, thinner less occlusive moisturizer formulations (e.g., Epidermal Repair by SkinCeuticals or ReBalance by PCA SKIN) with frequent application are preferable for managing dryness and pruritis.

Superficial abrasions can occur with aggressive MDA treatments, particularly in older patients and in thin-skinned areas. Abrasions typically appear as erythematous, slightly raised fine lines, which are commonly referred to as "striping". They may also be circular if the tip dwelled too long or excessive downward pressure was applied in one spot (with MDA devices that do not have recessed tips). Abrasions are not usually evident during treatment, but become visible immediately after treatment. After a few days, they may crust slightly and may hyperpigment. Abrasions and crusts are managed with moist wound care using a topical antibiotic ointment (e.g., bacitracin) daily and an adhesive dressing as needed until healed. Hyperpigmentation can be managed as outlined above.

Infections are extremely rare with MDA and require treatment specific to the pathogen. Activation of herpes simplex may occur despite adequate prophylactic antiviral medication use prior to treatment. Herpes simplex can be treated using a higher dose antiviral that is different from the prophylactic medication (e.g., valacyclovir 1 g twice per day for 7 days). Bacterial and fungal infections are extremely rare, but are possible any time the skin barrier is breached. The reader is referred to Complications in the Chemical Peels section for additional information on management of infections. It is advisable to culture infections if any there is a question of the diagnosis before initiating therapy. The reader is referred to Complications in the Chemical Peels section for additional information on management of infections.

Contact dermatitis may occur after MDA due to the products applied during or after treatment. This typically presents as prolonged erythema with small erythematous papules and can be treated with a low-potency steroid (e.g., hydrocortisone 2.5% or 1%) applied twice daily for 3–5 days.

Urticaria is a rare complication, and may be due to application of a vacuum to the skin, referred to as dermatographic or pressure-induced urticaria. Ice may be applied, an oral antihistamine (e.g., cetirizine 10 mg) given to the patient, and a high-potency topical steroid used in-office to the treatment area (e.g., triamcinolone 0.5%) and the patient sent home with a low-potency steroid (see above).

Petechiae and **purpura** can occur with overly aggressive vacuum settings, particularly in older patients, thin-skinned areas, and with anticoagulant use. Petechiae, visible as pin-point red dots, typically resolve in 3–5 days and purpura, typically visible as a circular red bruise, can take up to 2 weeks to clear.

Scarring is remotely possible and might be seen with the use of aggressive treatment parameters, particularly if infection occurs or crusts are excoriated. **Hypopigmentation** is also a possibility, and is usually temporary but may be permanent.

Notes on Specific Lesions and Conditions

- **Seborrheic keratoses (SKs)**. MDA can reduce the hyperkeratosis of SKs but does not usually improve the associated hyperpigmentation.
- **Actinic keratoses (AKs)**. MDA (without PDT) is not a treatment for AKs as the rough texture of these lesions may be their only presenting sign. AKs have a small potential for conversion to squamous cell carcinoma, therefore, and treatment of AKs with appropriate therapies is recommended.
- **Nevi**. Moles cannot be removed with MDA due to the depth of the melanocytes. Attempted removal may depigment moles and possibly result in scarring.
- **Erythematous conditions such as rosacea, telangiectasia, and Poikiloderma of Civatte**. Treatment of erythematous conditions with MDA is controversial. Clearly, excessive vacuum pressures can accentuate erythema. However, patients with rosacea, for example, have impaired barrier function and mild MDA treatments performed with low vacuum settings may strengthen the epidermal barrier, ultimately reducing skin sensitivity and erythema. Some providers, therefore, do perform MDA on patients with erythematous conditions using reduced vacuum settings in areas of high vascularity such as the midface and chin, and higher settings around the periphery of the face.
- **Acne**. MDA may be used for comedonal acne and mild-to-moderate papulopustular acne. However, it is advisable to avoid pustules. Alternative treatments for severe papulopustular acne such as oral medications and/or chemical peels are preferred treatment options.

Combining Aesthetic Treatments

Enhanced results, whether treating sun-damaged skin or other skin conditions, can be achieved when MDA is combined with other skin care treatments discussed in this practical guide, including chemical peels and daily skin care products. MDA can also be safely combined with other minimally invasive aesthetic procedures such as lasers and intense pulsed light devices, or with injectable procedures (see Combination Therapies in the Introduction and Foundation Concepts section for additional information about combining MDA with other treatments).

Reimbursement and Financial Considerations

Microdermabrasion is not reimbursed by insurance. Charges for treatments vary widely and are largely determined by local prices. Patients may pay for individual treatments, which typically range from $100 to $175. However, as MDA results are cumulative, a series of treatments (usually six) may be offered so that patients achieve the best possible results with the greatest satisfaction.

CPT Codes

- 17999, unlisted skin procedure
- A9270, non-covered service (for non-Medicare carriers)

In 2008, the American Academy of Dermatology clarified that CPT Code 15783 (dermabrasion, superficial, any site) is not appropriate to use for MDA.

ICD-9 Codes

- 706.1   Acne vulgaris
- 709.09   Melasma
- 709.0   Dyschromia, unspecified
- 701.8   Wrinkling of skin
- 709.2   Scarring

Topical Skin Care Products

Topical skin care products are used to treat photoaged skin and other dermatologic conditions such as facial erythema, acne, and hyperpigmentation. Improvements are cumulative and typically require 3–6 months of consistent use to become evident. Results for most skin conditions can be accelerated and enhanced by combining topical products with chemical peel and microdermabrasion exfoliation treatments. Topical products are also commonly used to support results of other minimally invasive aesthetic procedures such as lasers and intense pulsed light therapies.

Topical products range from prescription and over-the-counter (OTC) drugs that contain active ingredients to affect the structure and function of skin, to cosmetic products that alter the appearance of skin. Cosmeceuticals lie within this spectrum, and may be defined as either OTC products or cosmetics that deliver perceptible skin benefits. Cosmeceuticals are not recognized as a product category by the U.S. Food and Drug Administration (FDA), and therefore, are not routinely evaluated for safety or efficacy. They are, however, one of the fastest growing areas of aesthetic medicine and represent a multibillion dollar industry. Due to the plethora of products available and limited number of peer-reviewed studies, incorporating cosmeceuticals into treatment plans can be challenging. The following section provides a basic foundation in cosmeceutical ingredients to assist with decision-making when using cosmeceuticals for the treatment of photoaged skin and other common aesthetic skin conditions. This book also endeavors to be practical, and specific examples of products that may be used as part of regimens are also given in the following section. Many alternative products are equally appropriate and these examples are merely included as a convenience to assist providers in getting started with incorporating products into daily practice.

Treatment of Photoaged Skin

This section focuses on a targeted group of topical skin care products used for treatment and prevention of photoaging, referred to as the Topical Product Regimen for Photoaged Skin (see below). These rejuvenation products, consisting primarily of cosmeceuticals, can be readily combined with superficial chemical peels and/or microdermabrasion treatments to accelerate and enhance results. Products used for treatment address several aspects of the aging process, including stimulation of skin exfoliation and epidermal renewal, increase synthesis of collagen and other dermal matrix components, evening skin coloration (i.e., skin tone), and improving hydration. Products used for prevention of photoaging protect against damage from free radicals and ultraviolet radiation. These goals can be accomplished using rejuvenation products in three simple steps: cleanse, treat, and protect. General guidelines for the use of topical products are reviewed below and providers are advised to follow manufacturer instructions for each specific product.

Cleanse

This first step of the Topical Product Regimen prepares the skin for the subsequent application of topical treatment products. An effective cleanser thoroughly removes dirt,

Topical Product Regimen for Photoaged Skin

Steps	Purpose	Product Type	Example Products with Key Ingredients (Brand Name and Manufacturer)
Cleanse	Remove surface debris and sebum	Gentle facial cleanser	For example, Cream cleanser (Creamy Cleanser by PCA SKIN or Gentle Cleanser by SkinCeuticals)
Treat	Accelerate epidermal regeneration	Growth factor	For example, NouriCel-MD (TNS Recovery Complex by SkinMedica) or PSP (BIO-SERUM by NEOCUTIS)
	Regulate cellular turnover	Retinoid	For example, Retinol 1% (by SkinCeuticals) or retinol 1% with retinyl palmitate 0.1% and retinyl acetate 0.1% (Tri-retinol Complex by SkinMedica)
	Maintain hydration levels	Moisturizer	For example, Panthenol and mango butter-based cream with oils of grape seed, rose hip, and macademia (Emollience by SkinCeuticals) or petrolatum-based cream with dimethicone, sweet almond oil and tocopherol acetate (Cetaphil Cream by Galderma).
Protect	Prevent cellular oxidation	Antioxidant	For example, L-ascorbic acid 15% with alpha tocopherol 1% and ferulic acid (CE Ferulic by SkinCeuticals) or L-ascorbic acid 20% (Professional-C Serum by Obagi)
	Prevent damage from UV radiation	Sunscreen	For example, Titanium dioxide 7.3% with zinc oxide 3.4% (Daily Physical Defense SPF 30 by SkinMedica) or zinc oxide 7% with octinoxate 7.5% (Ultimate UV Defense SPF 30 by SkinCeuticals)

A limited number of products are listed as examples and many other products are equally appropriate. This Regimen is indicated for patients with normal to dry skin.

oil, makeup and other debris as well as desquamated corneocytes and microorganisms, yet is gentle enough to not strip the skin of its natural lipids.

- **Soap** is highly alkaline with a pH of about 11 and can disrupt the skin's pH causing barrier dysfunction, irritation, and dryness. A properly formulated gentle daily cleanser has a pH close to the skin's pH of 4.5–6.0.
- **Toners** consist of ingredients such as alcohol or witch hazel that remove the skin's natural oils. While they may be of benefit for acneic skin, they are rarely necessary for photoaged skin that tends to be drier. In addition, toners are commonly used following soaps to restore the skin's pH, and are not necessary when using a pH-balanced cleanser.

- **Surfactants** are foaming agents that are included in some products to enhance removal of surface oils and leave patients with a "squeaky clean" feeling after cleansing. Commonly used surfactants include sodium and ammonium laurel sulfate, sodium laureth sulfate, cocamidopropyl betaine, and lauroamphocarboxyglycinate. Foaming cleansers are more drying and are favored for oily and acneic skin. When treating photoaged skin, a cream-based cleanser which does not foam is a good option.

Cleanser Application (e.g., Creamy Cleanser by PCA SKIN)

1. Apply a dime-sized amount of cleanser to moistened face.
2. Massage cleanser thoroughly with fingertips.
3. Rinse with warm water and pat dry.
4. Cleanse twice daily.

Treat

The second step in the Topical Product Regimen for the Photoaged Skin involves stimulating exfoliation and epidermal renewal, increasing synthesis of dermal collagen and other matrix components, evening skin tone, and improving hydration. A single product usually contains several ingredients and so, multiple functions can be addressed with a limited number of products. Product consistency determines the order in which they are applied. The thinnest product is applied first, and the thickest last (e.g., gel, then serum, then lotion, and finally cream).

Growth Factors

Fibroblast growth factor products contain fibroblast secreted substances such as epidermal growth factor, transforming growth factor beta and platelet-derived growth factor, all of which stimulate fibroblast synthesis of collagen production and other extracellular matrix (ECM) components. Growth factor products may be obtained from a variety of sources, including fibroblasts in neonatal human foreskin or recombinant human epidermal growth factor engineered by yeast and bacteria. Twice daily application for 3 months of a growth factor product containing human growth factors, cytokines, and natural proteins (TNS Recovery Complex by SkinMedica) has been shown to improve skin hydration and reduce roughness, hyperpigmentation, and wrinkles in photoaged skin. When treating photoaged skin, a growth factor product is recommended as part of the Topical Product Regimen.

   Kinetin (N6-furfuryladenine) is a naturally occurring plant cytokine which is an antioxidant. It also functions as a fibroblast growth factor on cultured human fibroblast cells, but there is limited in vivo data on clinical efficacy.

Growth Factor Application (e.g., TNS Recovery Complex by SkinMedica)

1. Apply 1 pump of product every evening after the skin is cleansed.
2. Increase application frequency to twice daily if desired.

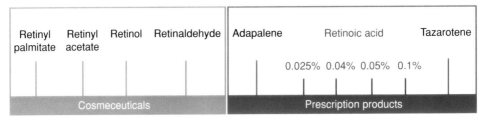

FIGURE 1 ● Topical retinoids.

Retinoids

Retinoids are vitamin A derivatives and analogs which range from potent prescription products such as tretinoin and synthetic tretinoin derivatives such as tazarotene, to less active cosmeceutical products such as retinol and retinaldehyde (Fig. 1). Retinoids promote healthy epidermal turn over and proper skin function through reducing corneocyte cohesion and enhancing desquamation, inhibiting melanogenesis, antioxidant functions, stimulating collagen production, and reducing keratinization within hair follicles (i.e., clogged pores). They are effective for treatment of photoaged skin as well as hyperpigmentation and acne. Due to their stimulating effects, it is advisable to use caution with retinoids in patients with rosacea or sensitive skin, as erythema can be exacerbated.

Prescription retinoids have the most profound and rapid rejuvenating effects on photoaged skin. Benefits are usually apparent by 1 month with improved texture due to compaction of the stratum corneum, and by 3 months reduction of hyperpigmentation and fine lines are visible. Prescription-strength retinoids can be used alone or in combination with other products, such as the Obagi Nu-Derm group of products which includes a prescription retinoid, alpha hydroxy acids, hydroquinone, and sunscreen. A significant disadvantage to prescription retinoids is "retinoid dermatitis" associated with their use consisting of erythema, sensitivity, and skin flaking. While this irritative response spontaneously resolves for most patients after 4–6 weeks of use, it can persist for longer. In addition, combining prescription retinoids with other in-office aesthetic procedures such as lasers and chemical peels can be challenging. Prescription retinoids are discontinued 1–2 weeks prior to procedures to allow for an intact epidermis at the time of treatment, and are restarted 1–2 weeks after procedures. This repeated stopping and starting cyclically can induce retinoid dermatitis. Therefore, prescription retinoids are often used as a stand-alone intervention for photoaged skin, as opposed to integrating them into treatment plans with other minimally invasive procedures.

Cosmeceutical retinoids are less effective than prescription retinoids in reducing the signs of photoaging; however, they rarely cause retinoid dermatitis when used in recommended doses and are well tolerated by patients. Retinol is one of the most commonly used cosmeceutical retinoids for photoaging and is an important component of the Topical Product Regimen for Photoaged Skin. Cosmeceutical retinoids are converted to the active form of retinoic acid after application to the skin as follows:

Retinol esters ↔ Retinol → Retinaldehyde → Retinoic acid
  (Storage form)   (Active form)

Cosmeceutical Retinoids

- **Retinaldehyde** is an immediate precursor to retinoic acid. It requires stabilization to remain in an active form in skin care products.

- **Retinol** is the most commonly used cosmeceutical form of vitamin A. New stabilizing technologies such as polymers and antioxidant additives have made it possible to have more active and effective retinol topical products.
- **Retinol esters** have weaker biologic activity.
  - **Retinyl palmitate** is the ester of retinol and palmitic acid, and is the primary storage form of vitamin A. It is typically used for its antioxidant properties in sunscreen and moisturizer products.
  - **Retinyl acetate** is the ester of retinol with acetic acid.
  - **Retinyl propionate** is the ester of retinol and propionic acid.

Retinoid Application (e.g., Retinol 1% by SkinCeuticals)

1. Apply a small pea-sized amount every third evening for 2 weeks.
2. Increase application frequency to every other evening for 2 weeks.
3. Increase application frequency to every evening as tolerated.
   - Flaking is normal and expected as is a mild pink color to the skin.
4. Apply in the evening.

If prescribing **tretinoin** (e.g., Retin-A), the above general guidelines can also be followed with a starting dose of 0.5 g of retinoic acid 0.025–0.05%. One gram of a cream is roughly equivalent to 1 inch of most products squeezed from an average sized tube, and 0.5 g is ½ inch. Skin redness, flaking, and sensitivity are anticipated when using prescription-strength retinoids. Tolerability can be increased by mixing tretinoin in equal parts with the evening moisturizer; however, this may reduce efficacy.

Moisturizers

Moisturizers enhance epidermal barrier function and hydrate the epidermis by increasing flux of water from the dermis to the epidermis and by reducing evaporative water loss. Skin is rendered more supple and healthy with the use of moisturizers, and clinically demonstrates improvements in smoothness and wrinkles. These effects can be temporary, visible only while the moisturizer is present, or can also be long-lasting when the integrity of the skin barrier is strengthened following repeated use.

There are three main types of ingredients in moisturizers (occlusives, humectants, and emollients), each of which serves a different function (see Table 1). Petrolatum is one of the most occlusive agents; however, it is poorly tolerated due to its sticky consistency and is usually combined with silicone or mineral oil to improve its consistency. Light oils such as evening primrose and borage seed oils are mild occlusives and, in addition to their anti-inflammatory properties, also function as moisturizers. Glycerin is an effective humectant; however, it also has an undesirable consistency which can be improved by combining it with other humectants such as panthenol and sodium pyrrolidone carbonic acid (PCA). Hyaluronic acid is a commonly used humectant, as is sodium hyaluronate, a salt of hyaluronic acid that has increased skin penetration compared to hyaluronic acid. The term "emollient" is sometimes used interchangeably with "moisturizer"; however, it is one of the components found in moisturizers and has

TABLE 1

Moisturizer Ingredients and Their Function

Moisturizer Type	Function	Ingredients
Occlusives	Trap water on the skin surface and enhance lipid component of epidermal barrier	• Oils (e.g., petrolatum, mineral oil) • Cholesterol, squalene • Waxes (e.g., beeswax, carnauba wax, liquid wax) • Silicones (e.g., dimethicone, cyclomethicone) • Stearic acid, detyl alcohol, stearyl alcohol • Lanolin, lanolin alcohol • Shea butter (Butyrospermum parkii)
Humectants	Attract water from the dermis into the epidermis	• Glycerin • Urea • Hyaluronic acid and sodium hyaluronate • Sorbitol • Sodium pyrrolidone carboxylic acid (PCA) • Propylene glycol • Panthenol (provitamin B5)
Emollients	Smooth roughened epidermis	• C12–15 alkyl benzoate • Cetyl stearate • Glyceryl stearate • Octyl octanoate • Decyl oleate • Isostearyl alcohol

a specific function to fill in gaps between desquamating corneocytes to enhance skin smoothness. Most moisturizers are composed of all three ingredient types in a product that is cosmetically elegant which does not feel greasy or sticky.

Moisturizers are formulated as emulsions of oil and water, and their consistency depends on the relative amounts of oil and water. Ointments are the thickest moisturizers and contain nearly all oil (80% oil and 20% water). They are most useful for extremely dry or chaffed skin and are not meant for prolonged use as this may precipitate acne. Creams contain approximately equal parts of oil and water, making them thinner than ointments but thicker than lotions. Lotions, often referred to as light moisturizers, contain more water than oil. Serums are comprised almost entirely of water. Gels are water-based emulsions, and are the lightest of the moisturizers. They penetrate the skin quickly, leaving no residue on the skin's surface, and are well suited for patients with acne prone or oily skin.

The following list shows moisturizer vehicle formulations in descending order of thickness:

- Ointment (thickest)
- Cream
- Lotion
- Serum
- Gel (thinnest)

Moisturizers function as ideal vehicles for delivery of functional ingredients to the skin as they are formulated with both oil and water, and can contain both hydrophilic and lipophilic ingredients. The key functional ingredients included in a moisturizer also have an impact on a product's overall moisturizing capabilities. For example, although serums are inherently less hydrating, when they contain hydrating active ingredients (such as panthenol, evening primrose, or borage seed oils) they can improve barrier function and may provide hydration equivalent to a cream.

Moisturizer Application

1. Select the appropriate moisturizer based on the patient's skin type.
2. If using creams in jars, dispense the product with a disposable applicator such as a cotton-tipped applicator (i.e., Q-tip).
   - A recent study found that products repeatedly inoculated with fingers cultured positive for streptococcus and staphylococcus bacteria and fungi.
3. A thick cream moisturizer may also be applied sparingly in the periocular area on top of a facial moisturizer for additional hydration.
   - Application of excessive product in the periocular area can cause ocular irritation.
4. Apply in the evening after other thinner topical products (such as serums and gels) and if needed, in the morning after an antioxidant and before a sunscreen.

Other Treatment Products for Photoaged Skin

Exfoliants

Most chemical exfoliants function by breaking intercellular corneodesmosomal bonds in the stratum corneum, which promotes desquamation (i.e., exfoliation). Removal of the outer skin layers thins the stratum corneum, stimulates epidermal renewal, and evens out the distribution of melanin in photoaged skin. This is clinically evident as improved skin smoothness and reduced hyperpigmentation and fine lines. Use of exfoliant products may also facilitate penetration and efficacy of other topical products in a regimen.

Exfoliants can be incorporated into the Topical Product Regimen for Photoaged Skin once patients' skin has acclimated to the initial Regimen. They are usually applied daily in the evening. Some exfoliants, such as glycolic acid, can be irritating and application may be initiated every other evening for 2 weeks and then advanced to every evening. Overuse of exfoliants, which can occur if exfoliant ingredients are constituents in multiple products, can impair the skin barrier resulting in chronic irritation and erythema.

- **Alpha hydroxy acids (AHAs)** are derived primarily from fruit acids and include glycolic (sugar cane), malic (apples), tartaric (grapes), citric (citrus), mandelic (almonds), lactic (milk) and phytic (rice) acids. In addition to the epidermal benefits listed above, skin treated with AHAs also shows improved hydration and histologically demonstrates benefits in the dermis with improved elastin fiber quality and increased deposition of glycosaminoglycans and collagen. Glycolic, lactic, citric, and mandelic acids are commonly used for treatment of photoaged skin, in concentrations less than 10%. AHAs are also used as chemical peel agents where they are formulated with higher concentrations in more acidic preparations. Lactic acid is one of the most hydrating AHAs and is often used for dry skin types. Polyhydroxy acids (such as gluconolactone) and bionic acids (such as lactobionic acid and maltobionic acid) are second generation hydroxy acids that have AHA-like effects but are less irritating, and can be used for sensitive skin. They also have humectant and antioxidant properties.

- **Beta hydroxy acids (BHAs)** include salicylic acid. Salicylic acid (SA) is derived from willow tree bark, wintergreen oil, and sweet birch. It is lipophilic, unlike AHAs which are water soluble, and readily penetrates and dissolves sebum making SA a highly effective therapy for acne. In addition, SA has anti-inflammatory effects which make it suitable for sensitive skin and rosacea. Concentrations up to 2% are commonly found in home care products. Capryloyl salicylic acid (also referred to as β-lipohydroxy acid or LHA) is the ester of salicylic acid and functions similarly to SA with increased lipophilicity.
- **Niacinamide (vitamin B3)** is a gentle exfoliant appropriate for sensitive skin that reduces inflammation.
- **Urea** exfoliates and hydrates skin. Urea functions as a humectant in lower concentrations (<10%) by increasing water binding sites on keratinocytes. In higher concentrations (>20%) it is an exfoliant. It is commonly used in concentrations of 5–25% in topical facial products.
- **Vigna aconitifolia seed extract** (mat bean) has mild exfoliant properties and stimulates collagen production.

Peptides

Peptides are short chains of amino acids that act as transmitters of information within the body. Those used for skin care are categorized as neurotransmitter modulating peptides, carrier peptides, or signal peptides. In photoaged skin, topical peptides are primarily used for improving skin texture and fine lines. Peptide products are well tolerated and may be applied daily in the morning and evening. The topical use of peptides is still relatively new and there is limited data on efficacy.

- **Neurotransmitter-modulating peptides** include **acetyl hexapeptide-8** (e.g., Argireline by Lipotec). Acetyl hexapeptide-8 is designed to reduce muscle contraction by inhibiting acetylcholine release. One study found that, when applied twice daily for 1 month, acetyl hexapeptide-8 reduced the depth of dynamic wrinkles.
- **Carrier peptides** include **copper** peptides. Topical products with carrier peptides deliver metals such as copper to the skin where they are used as cofactors in enzymatic reactions involving antioxidants, and production of collagen, elastin, and glycosaminoglycans.
- **Signal peptides** act as protein mimics to stimulate synthesis of collagen and other dermal matrix components.
  - **Palmitoyl pentapeptide-4** (e.g., Matrixyl by Sederma, StriVectin by Klein Becker) is a pro-collagen peptide sequence that stimulates the production of collagen and fibronectin.
  - **Palmitoyl oligopeptide** (e.g., by Sederma) is derived from elastin and stimulates growth of fibroblasts and blood vessels.

Matrix Metalloproteinase (MMP) Inhibitors

Matrix metalloproteinases (MMPs) are naturally occurring enzymes that degrade the skin's ECM and facilitate the recycling of spent collagen, elastin, and glycosaminoglycans. In young healthy skin, production of matrix components exceeds destruction caused by MMPs. In photoaged skin, matrix degradation is accelerated as MMP activity is upregulated by UV light. Accelerated matrix degradation combined with age-related decline in collagen synthesis, decreases the structural integrity of the skin's matrix and contributes to formation of wrinkles, skin laxity, and telangiectasias.

MMP inhibitors such as lactobionic acid, resveratrol, epigallocatechin gallate (EGCG), and idebenone protect against degradation of the dermal matrix. They also increase dermal collagen and elastin and clinically improve textural changes in photoaged skin. MMP inhibitors are typically well tolerated and may be used daily in the morning or evening.

Amino Sugars

N-acetylglucosamine, an amino sugar, is a component of hyaluronic acid. Topical application has been shown to stimulate synthesis of hyaluronic acid in fibroblasts and keratinocytes, increase skin thickness, and enhance exfoliation. Clinically, N-acetylglucosamine reduces wrinkles and hyperpigmentation, and increases hydration.

Protect

Most of the changes seen with skin aging are due to harmful effects from years of cumulative UV exposure. The third step in the Topical Product Regimen for Photoaged Skin involves protection of the skin from UV-induced cutaneous damage.

Antioxidants

Ultraviolet light generates destructive free radicals in skin which oxidize nucleic acids, proteins, and lipids, leading to the development of skin cancers and signs of photoaging. Topical antioxidants protect the skin from free radical damage and provide added support to the body's own endogenous antioxidant capabilities. Antioxidants can donate an electron to the radical and thereby act as a reducing agent (primary antioxidant), chelate metal ions and thereby remove potential radical initiators (secondary antioxidant), or facilitate the antioxidant activity of other compounds (coantioxidants). Commonly used topical antioxidants are shown in Table 2 and discussed below. Vitamins C and E are some of the most effective and most widely used topical antioxidants. In addition to their photoprotective capabilities, vitamins C and E also treat photoaged skin by reducing wrinkles through increasing dermal collagen, and they have anti-inflammatory properties. Vitamin C also reduces hyperpigmentation through inhibition of melanin synthesis. When treating photoaged skin, a product containing vitamins C and E in serum form is incorporated into the Topical Product Regimen.

- **Vitamin C** is a water-soluble antioxidant that protects the skin's aqueous components. It is highly effective in the **L-ascorbic acid** form, with a pH of 3.5 or less, in concentrations of 10–20%. L-acsorbic acid is also formulated in a stabilized anhydrous base in some products. After oral administration, L-ascorbic acid is excreted by the kidneys and the skin does not "see" adequate concentrations of L-ascorbic acid. L-ascorbic acid must, therefore, be administered topically to have therapeutic benefits in skin.
- **Vitamin E** is a lipid-soluble antioxidant that protects cell membranes and the stratum corneum from oxidative stress. **Alpha tocopherol** and **tocotrienol** are the most potent forms of vitamin E. Other forms used in topical products include vitamin E esters, such as tocopherol acetate and tocopherol palmitate. Vitamins C and E work synergistically as coantioxidants to increase the bioavailablity of one another.
- Many other vitamin and botanical antioxidant ingredients are used in rejuvenation products (Table 2). Some antioxidants have multiple effects on skin such as algae extracts which also function as humectants, and niacinamide which is also an exfoliant.

TABLE 2

Antioxidant Topical Products

Antioxidant	Source
Beta-carotene (provitamin A)	Carrots, broccoli, spinach, peaches, apricots
Caffeine	Coffeeberry, tea, cocoa beans
Coffea arabica extract	Coffeeberry
Epigallocatechin gallate (EGCG)	Green tea
Ergothioneine	Red and black beans, specialty mushrooms
Ferulic acid	Tomatoes, sweet corn, rice bran, oranges, carrots
Glutathione (GSH)	Avocado, asparagus, garlic, tomatoes, raw eggs
Idebenone	Coenzyme Q10 derivative (engineered)
Kinetin (N6-furfuryladenine)	Plant parts and yeast
L-ascorbic acid (vitamin C)	Dark leafy greens, citrus fruits, colored berries
Lipoic acid (alpha lipoic acid, ALA, thioctic acid)	Spinach, broccoli, yeast, rice bran
Melatonin	Fruits, vegetables, cereals
Niacinamide (vitamin B3)	Niacin
Panthenol (provitamin B5, pantothenic acid)	Whole grains, legumes, meat, eggs
Phloretin	Apple tree leaves
Polyphenolic fruit extracts (polyphenols)	Dark red fruits and berries, apples, grapes, pears
Polyphenolic vegetable extracts (polyphenols)	Onion, broccoli, cabbage, celery, red vegetables
Resveratrol	Colored berries, grapes, red wine, peanut plant
Silymarin flavonoids (e.g., silybin and silydianin)	Milk thistle plant
Soy flavonoids (e.g., genistein and daidzein)	Soy
Superoxide dismutase (SOD)	Melons, wheat, corn, soy
Tocopherol (vitamin E)	Vegetable oils, corn, soybeans, wheat germ, tree nut oils
Ubiquinone	Coenzyme Q10 derivative
Verbascoside	Lilac leaf

Antioxidant Application (e.g., CE Ferulic by SkinCeuticals)

1. Dispense 3–5 drops of serum and rub onto the entire face (excluding eyelids) using both hands after the skin is cleansed.
2. Wait a few minutes for absorption.
   * If the skin feels tacky reduce the quantity applied subsequently.
3. Apply in the morning daily.
   * Certain antioxidant formulations may be applied to eyelids if indicated by the manufacturer (e.g., AOX Eye Gel by SkinCeuticals).

Sunscreens

Sunscreens protect against UV-induced cutaneous damage by reducing exposure to UV radiation. A broad-spectrum sunscreen, offering protection from both UVA and UVB radiation, is an essential component of The Topical Product Regimen for Photoaged Skin.

- **Ultraviolet B radiation** (UVB, 290–320 nm), commonly referred to as the burning rays, are short wavelengths of light that are absorbed by the epidermis. These rays are strongest from 10 AM to 4 PM.
- **Ultraviolet A radiation** (UVA, 320–400 nm), commonly referred to as the aging rays, are long wavelengths of light that penetrate into the dermis. These penetrating rays breakdown collagen and elastin and are primarily responsible for fine lines and wrinkles. Unlike UVB rays, UVA rays' strength remains constant throughout the day and UVA rays travel through glass.

There are two main types of sunscreen ingredients each of which has a different mechanism of action. **Physical sunscreens**, composed of inorganic compounds, reflect, scatter and to some degree, absorb UV light. **Chemical sunscreens**, composed of organic sunscreens, absorb UV light. Figure 2 shows common sunscreen ingredients and their UV blocking capabilities.

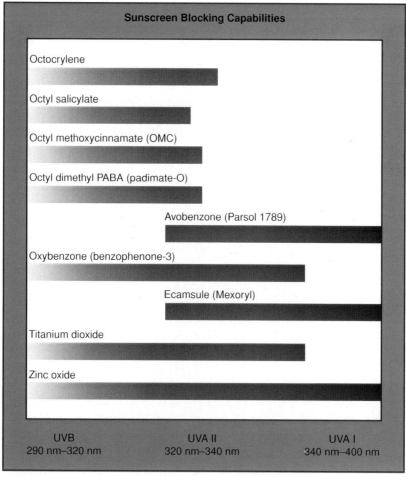

FIGURE 2 ● Sunscreens and their ultraviolet blocking properties.

Effective sunscreen products are broad-spectrum, maintain stability when exposed to sunlight, and have an appealing consistency that promotes everyday use. Most broad-spectrum sunscreens combine multiple organic and inorganic sunscreen ingredients within one product and usually contain at least one of the following for UVA protection: zinc oxide, titanium dioxide, stabilized avobenzone, or ecamsule (Mexoryl).

Sun protection factor (SPF) indicates the level of UVB protection of a sunscreen product. Currently, providers' knowledge of the UVA blocking capabilities of individual sunscreen ingredients is necessary to determine a product's UVA coverage. New labeling including indications for broad-spectrum coverage and redefinition of SPF as Sunburn Protection Factor has been mandated by the FDA.

Photostability of sunscreen products is determined by the ingredients and formulation. For example, avobenzone alone has poor photostability. However, the addition of other agents such as octinoxate, titanium dioxide, or oxybenzone (i.e., HelioPlex) renders avobenzone photostable. Sunscreens that have the Skin Cancer Foundation's "Seal of Recommendation" have all undergone testing and passed standards for photostability, SPF determination, phototoxicity, and contact irritancy.

Sunscreen Application (e.g., Daily Physical Defense SPF 30 by SkinMedica)

1. Apply a broad-spectrum sunscreen with SPF 30 or greater after cleansing the skin and applying an antioxidant.
   - For the face apply $1/3$ tsp (1.5 mL).
   - For the upper chest (i.e., décolletage) apply $1/3$ tsp (1.5 mL).
   - For the anterior and posterior neck apply $1/3$ tsp (1.5 mL).
   - It is important to note that studies looking at the quantity of sunscreens applied show that most patients apply 25% of the recommended amount. With this quantity, an SPF 30 product only offers SPF 2 protection.
2. Rub minimally during application.
   - Excessively rubbing sunscreens that contain zinc and titanium can result in increased white coloration of the product which is unsightly.
3. Apply sunscreens daily, in the morning.
4. For outdoor activities, apply sunscreen to all sun exposed areas prior to activity. Coverage of the whole body requires 30 mL (or one shot glass). Areas commonly missed include: ears, temples, neck and tops of feet. Reapply (the above amounts) after 2 hours or immediately after swimming or perspiring. Water resistant sunscreens can be effective for either 40 minutes or 80 minutes in water and will be labeled as such when the new labeling guidelines are in effect.

Results

Visible improvements in photoaged skin with the use of topical products are typically evident over 3–6 months with regular use. Improved texture and brightness may be apparent by 1 month, and reduction of fine lines and hyperpigmentation by 3 months. These changes can be seen more rapidly with prescription products than with cosmeceutical products.

Figure 3 shows photoaged skin with wrinkling before (A) and after (B) daily use for 3 months of acetyl hexapeptide-8, epidermal growth factor, L-ascorbic acid 15%,

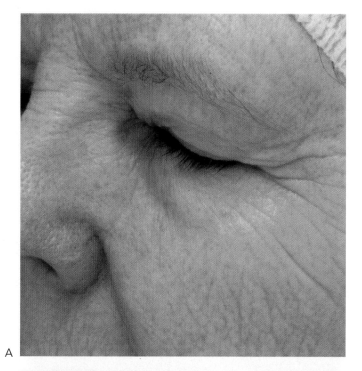

A

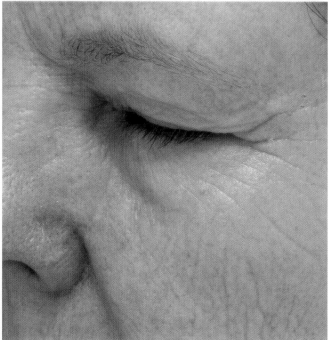

B

FIGURE 3 ● Photoaged skin with wrinkling before **(A)** and after **(B)**
daily use for 3 months of acetyl hexapeptide-8 and epigallocatechin
gallate (ExLinea Peptide Smoothing Serum), growth factor (Rejuvenating Serum), L-ascorbic acid 15% (C-Quench Antioxidant), retinol 1% with
Vigna aconitifolia seed extract 3% (Retinol Renewal with RestorAtive
Complex), palmitoyl pentapeptide-4 eye cream (EyeXcellence), shea
butter moisturizer (Collagen Hydrator), and a broad-spectrum sunscreen
of SPF 30. (Courtesy of PCA SKIN)

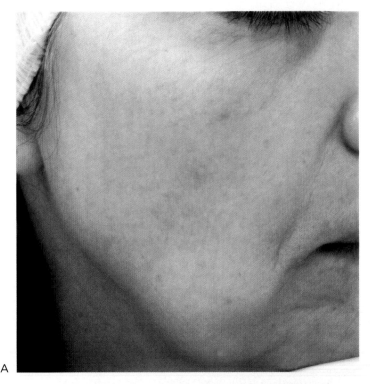

A

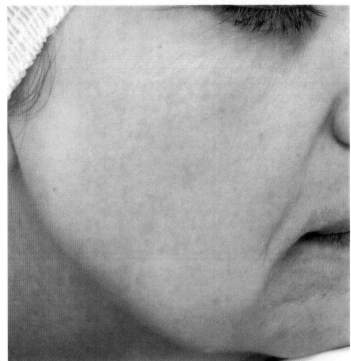

B

FIGURE 4 ● Photoaged skin with wrinkling and laxity before **(A)** and after **(B)** daily use for 2 months of retinol 1% with Vigna aconitifolia seed extract 3% (Retinol Renewal with RestorAtive Complex), soy flavonoid–based cream moisturizer (Après Peel Hydrating Balm), and a broad-spectrum sunscreen of SPF 30. (Courtesy of PCA SKIN)

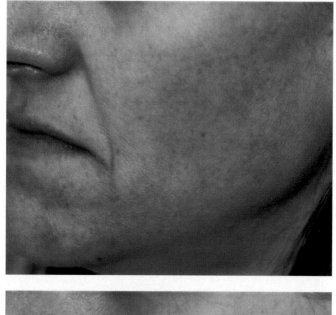

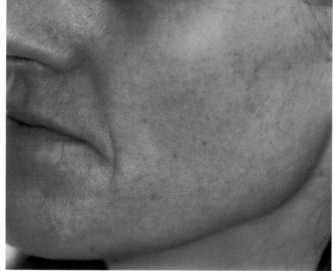

FIGURE 5 ● Photoaged skin with UV-induced hyperpigmentation before **(A)** and after **(B)** daily use for 3 months of tretinoin 0.05% (Retin-A), hydroquinone 4% (Clear), glycolic acid 6% with lactic acid 4% (Exfoderm Forte), and a broad-spectrum sunscreen of SPF 35 (Healthy Skin Protection). (Courtesy of Rebecca Small, MD)

retinol 1%, Vigna aconitifolia seed extract 3%, palmitoyl pentapeptide-4 eye cream, shea butter-based moisturizer and a broad-spectrum sunscreen of SPF 30.

Figure 4 shows photoaged skin with wrinkling and laxity before (A) and after (B) daily use for 2 months of retinol 1%, Vigna aconitifolia seed extract 3%, soy flavonoid-based moisturizer and a broad-spectrum sunscreen of SPF 30.

Figure 5 shows UV-induced hyperpigmentation before (A) and after (B) daily use for 3 months of tretinoin 0.05%, hydroquinone 4%, glycolic acid 6% with lactic acid 4% and a broad-spectrum sunscreen of SPF 30.

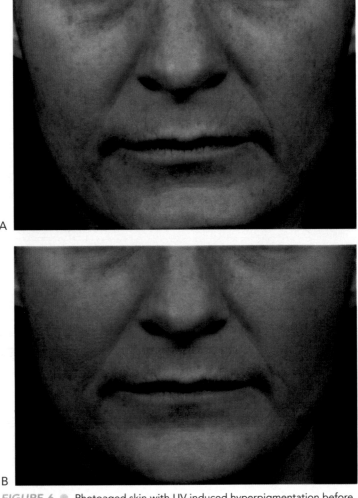

FIGURE 6 ● Photoaged skin with UV-induced hyperpigmentation before **(A)** and after **(B)** daily use for 2 months of retinol 1%, retinyl palmitate 0.1%, retinyl acetate 0.1% (Tri-retinol Complex), and a broad-spectrum sunscreen of SPF 30. (Courtesy of SkinMedica)

Figure 6 shows UV-induced hyperpigmentation before (A) and after (B) daily use for 2 months of retinol 1%, retinyl palmitate 0.1%, retinyl acetate 0.1% and a broad-spectrum sunscreen of SPF 30.

Figure 7 shows wrinkling before (A) and after (B) twice daily use for 6 months of growth factor and a broad-spectrum sunscreen of SPF 30.

Figure 8 shows darkened freckles and dullness before (A) and after (B) daily use for 6 weeks of hydroquinone 4%, L-ascorbic acid 10% with vitamin E, glycolic acid 7%, and a broad-spectrum sunscreen of SPF 30.

Common Follow-ups and Management

During the initial stages of implementing a Topical Product Regimen, it is advisable to have the patient return in 4–6 weeks to evaluate the skin, assess tolerability and adherence,

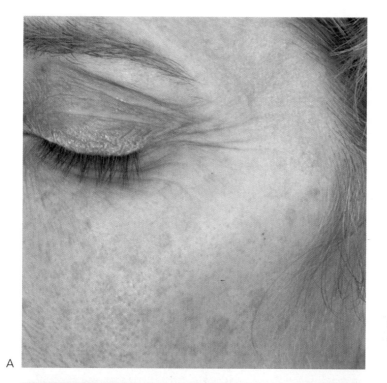

FIGURE 7 ● Photoaged skin with wrinkling before **(A)** and after **(B)** twice daily use for 6 months of growth factor (TNS Recovery Complex), and a broad-spectrum sunscreen of SPF 30. (Courtesy of SkinMedica)

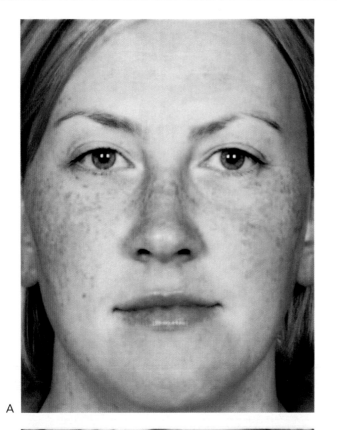

A

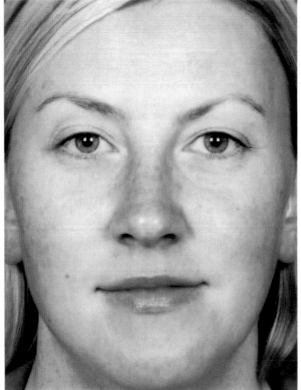

B

FIGURE 8 ● Photoaged skin with darkened freckles and dullness before **(A)** and after **(B)** daily use for 6 weeks of hydroquinone 4%, L-ascorbic acid 10% with vitamin E, glycolic acid 7%, and a broad-spectrum sunscreen of SPF 30 (Obagi-C Rx System). (Courtesy of Obagi)

and to make any necessary adjustments to their regimen. Providers may also inquire about dryness or oiliness and, although unlikely, assess for complications (see below).

- **Excessive dryness.** If skin is too dry, an additional hydrating product may be integrated into the regimen such as a hydrating serum (e.g., SkinCeutical's hydrating B5 gel that contains hyaluronic acid and vitamin B5 or PCA SKIN's Hydrating Serum that contains urea, sodium hyaluronate, niacinamide, and glycerin). The skin may also be exfoliated with in-office procedures such as microdermabrasion or a chemical peel to help treat dryness.
- **Excessive oiliness.** If the skin is too oily, the moisturizer may be changed to a thinner product such as a lotion or gel (e.g., SkinCeutical's Phyto Corrective Gel containing hyaluronic acid with thyme and cucumber extracts or PCA SKIN's ReBalance with borage seed and evening primrose oils, and aloe vera).
- **Subsequent follow-ups** once patients are satisfied with their skin care regimen are typically every 6 months or as needed to replenish products.

Enhancing Results for Photoaged Skin

If patients tolerate the Topical Product Regimen well, consider intensifying the regimen by adding an exfoliant product (e.g., SkinCeutical's Blemish and Age Defense containing AHAs and BHAs, or Obagi's Exfoderm which contains phytic acid or Exfoderm Forte which contains glycolic and lactic acids). Combining topical products with exfoliation treatments such as microdermabrasion and chemical peels also enhances results. In addition, other minimally invasive aesthetic procedures may also be used to enhance results for specific issues such as lasers and intense pulsed light for hyperpigmentation, erythema, and textural improvements; botulinum toxin for dynamic wrinkles and dermal fillers for static wrinkles, volume loss, and contour irregularities.

Topical Product Complications and Management

- Acne
- Milia
- Contact dermatitis
- Allergic reactions such as urticaria, and the remote possibility of severe reactions such as anaphylaxis
- Exacerbation of dermatoses such as seborrheic dermatitis, atopic dermatitis (eczema), and perioral dermatitis
- Exacerbation of erythema and skin sensitivity

Topical skin care products are generally very safe and well tolerated with minimal risks of complications. However, complications are possible with any therapy, and knowledge of these is important to minimize risks and help ensure the best possible results.

Acne flares are relatively common when starting new topical products, particularly in patients who are acne prone and, with the use of thicker products such as creams. Acne may develop within the first few weeks of new product use in patients with a strong history of acne, and in other patients may be delayed. Discontinuation of thick products is recommended with substitution for products that have a lighter consistency such as lotions, serums, or gels.

Milia are tiny 1–2 mm white papules that result from occlusion of sebaceous glands. Products with thick consistencies containing occlusive ingredients such as petrolatum can obstruct sebaceous glands and contribute to milia formation. Milia do not usually resolve spontaneously and require lancing with a 20 gauge needle and extraction (gentle squeezing with cotton-tipped applicators).

Contact dermatitis is one of the most common adverse reactions to topical products. Most forms of contact dermatitis are irritant in nature, as opposed to being truly allergic. Dermatitis reactions are usually mild and present with mild erythema, edema, and pruritis. The first step in management of any dermatitis is discontinuation of the offending product. Unfortunately, the offending product in a regimen is often unknown, and it is advisable to discontinue all topical products except for a gentle cleanser (such as Cetaphil Gentle Skin Cleanser by Galderma) and use a topical steroid for treatment. Mild to moderate dermatitis can be managed with application of a low potency corticosteroid cream (e.g., hydrocortisone 0.5–2.5%), and more intense eruptions with a medium potency (e.g., triamcinolone 0.1%) cream twice daily for 3–5 days or until the dermatitis resolves. Rarely, severe dermatitis reactions may occur that present with pronounced erythema, edema, and vesiculation within the treatment area and, if allergic in nature, can be remote from the site of application. A short course of oral steroids may be necessary in these cases (e.g., prednisone 20–40 mg/day tapered over 10 days) followed by topical steroids once the skin is intact if erythema persists.

Patients can develop dermatitis at any time to a product that was previously well tolerated. Limiting the use of potentially sensitizing ingredients such as fragrances can help prevent dermatitis. After the dermatitis has resolved, products may be reintroduced singly every 2–4 weeks, in an attempt to identify which product caused the reaction. Alternatively, a patch test may be performed whereby a small amount of product is placed discretely either behind the ear or on the underside of the forearm daily for 3–5 days, and the site evaluated for erythema and other signs of irritation. If a patch test is positive, that specific product is avoided. A negative patch test is reassuring and the product may be used; however, a negative test does not ensure that an adverse response will not occur.

Allergic reactions to topical products are rare. The most commonly encountered allergic reaction is urticaria, which responds to oral antihistamines (e.g., cetirizine 10 mg) and topical steroids (see above). There is a remote risk of severe systemic allergic reactions, such as bronchospasm or anaphylaxis necessitating emergency care. Salicylic acid is related to aspirin (acetylsalicylic acid) and, therefore, products containing salicylic acid should not be used on patients with a known aspirin allergy.

Exacerbation of dermatoses (such as seborrheic dermatitis, atopic dermatitis, and perioral dermatitis) or **exacerbation of erythema and skin sensitivity** can occur with the use of topical products that contain active ingredients. Using soothing products (see Treatment of Facial Erythema section below) and avoiding the more aggressive antiaging products such as hydroxy acids and retinoids can help reduce the likelihood of flaring these conditions.

Ingredients to Avoid or with Which to Use Caution

Cosmeceuticals are not regulated by the FDA and are therefore, not required to be evaluated for safety or efficacy. There are nearly 10,000 ingredients in cosmetic products most of which lack peer-reviewed clinical trials, making rigorous evaluation of products a challenge. The FDA website (www.fda.gov/Cosmetics/ProductandIngredientSafety) can aid in the evaluation of product safety. Below are a few examples of ingredients to avoid or with which to use caution:

- **Highly fragranced products** can be irritating to the skin.

- **Ascorbyl palmitate** is an ester comprised of ascorbic acid and palmitic acid. It is promoted as an antioxidant but may only have minimal efficacy. It does not have comparable effects to L-ascorbic acid, which is the only bioavailable form of vitamin C (such as collagen stimulation, epidermal thickening and pigment inhibition).
- **Phthalates** are esters of phthalic acid which are carriers for fragrances and softeners in some topical products, and are primarily used in plastics to increase flexibility. Phthalates are being removed from many products and packaging due to potential hormonal alterations and carcinogenicity.
- **Diethanolamine (DEA)** or **triethanolamine (TEA)** are used in products to produce a smooth consistency or lather. Both DEA and TEA may be harmless when alone, but when combined with other ingredients they can produce nitrosodiethanolamine, a known carcinogen.

Product Shelf Life

The shelf life of a topical product refers to the period of time that it remains effective and suitable for use. Once a product is exposed to oxygen, light, moisture, and external contamination, it develops microbial growth and rapidly degrades. Storing products in a cool, dry place out of direct sunlight, and dispensing with sanitary methods using applicators rather than fingers, can reduce microbial contamination and maintain a product's effectiveness. Preservatives are incorporated into products to help maintain shelf life. **Parabens** are common preservatives whose use is controversial. Some organizations such as the FDA have concluded that parabens are safe for use in cosmetic products. However, negative attention received in the media, due to concerns over possible estrogenic effects and association with cancer, has resulted in many manufacturers removing parabens from products. There are many other safe and effective preservatives available including phenoxyethanol, iodopropynyl butylcarbamate, and potassium sorbate. Retinol, vitamin C, and hydroquinone are particularly unstable products and if they turn brown in color or if vitamin C products crystallize, it is advisable to discard them.

Treatment of Facial Erythema: Rosacea and Sensitive Skin

Facial erythema is commonly seen in patients with rosacea, sensitive skin, and photoaged skin. Treatment is aimed at reducing inflammation and irritation, enhancing skin barrier function, increasing hydration, trigger avoidance, and sun protection. This section focuses on a targeted group of topical skin care products used for treatment and prevention of facial erythema, referred to as the Topical Product Regimen for Facial Erythema (see below). It includes nonirritating products that have low concentrations of active ingredients and excludes products containing fragrances and astringents. Many alternative selections of topical products are equally appropriate.

Cleanse

A cream-based nonfoaming cleanser is recommended to prevent further disruption of the barrier function.

● Topical Product Regimen for Facial Erythema: Rosacea and Sensitive Skin

Steps	Purpose	Product Type	Example Products with Key Ingredients (Brand Name and Manufacturer)
Cleanse	Remove surface debris and sebum	Gentle facial cleanser	For example, Cream cleanser (Creamy Cleanser by PCA SKIN or Gentle Cleanser by SkinCeuticals)
Treat	Reduce erythema	Anti-inflammatory and soothing	For example, Hyaluronic acid–based gel with thyme and cucumber extracts (Phyto Corrective Gel by SkinCeuticals) or dimethicone with algae and caperbud extracts (Anti-Redness Serum by PCA SKIN)
	Maintain hydration levels	Moisturizer	For example, Panthenol-based thin cream with borage and evening primrose oils and aloe vera (ReBalance by PCA SKIN) or glycerin-based lotion with panthenol, dimethicone and tocopheryl acetate (Cetaphil lotion by Galderma)
Protect	Prevent cellular oxidation	Antioxidant	For example, L-ascorbic acid 10% with ferulic acid 0.5%, and phloretin 2% serum (Phloretin CF by SkinCeuticals) or L-ascorbic acid 10% (Professional-C Serum by Obagi)
	Prevent damage from UV radiation	Sunscreen	For example, Titanium dioxide 7.3% with zinc oxide 3.4% (Daily Physical Defense SPF 30 by SkinMedica) or titanium dioxide 6% with zinc oxide 5% (Sheer Physical UV Defense SPF 50 by SkinCeuticals)

A limited number of products are listed as examples and many other products are equally appropriate. This Regimen is indicated for patients with normal to oily skin.

Treat

- **Light moisturizers** such as lotions, are one of the mainstays of therapy as they help restore healthy barrier function. Creams may also be used if the skin is dry and patients do not have acne (papulopustular) rosacea.
- **Soothing and anti-inflammatory** cosmeceutical ingredients (see Table 3) are either incorporated within a moisturizer product or into a separate product.
  - **Green tea** is a potent anti-inflammatory cosmeceutical due to its high concentration of polyphenols.
  - **Borage seed oil,** and to a lesser degree **evening primrose oil,** contains gamma-linolenic acid (GLA). GLA is converted to prostaglandin 1, which has potent anti-inflammatory effects on skin.
  - **Allantoin** and **bisabolol** are also commonly used in soothing topical products.
- **Azelaic acid** reduces erythema, treats acne papules associated with acne rosacea, and functions as a brightening agent. However, azelaic acid can be associated with a stinging sensation upon application and may not be well tolerated at higher percentages.
- **Mild exfoliants** such as niacinamide or less irritating polyhydroxy acids such as lactobionic acid may be used. Fruit acid exfoliants such as glycolic acid can exacerbate erythema and are usually avoided in patients with facial erythema.
- **Growth factors** are gentle enough to be used in patients with facial erythema. However, collagen stimulation is usually secondary to reduction of inflammation and these products are often incorporated after the initial topical product regimen is well established.

TABLE 3

Cosmeceuticals for Facial Erythema

Product	Function	Ingredient or Source
Algae extracts	Anti-inflammatory, angiogenesis inhibitor	Ascophyllum nodosum (brown) and Asparagopsis armata (red) algae
Allantoin	Soothing	Comfrey root or synthetically derived from uric acid
Aloe vera	Anti-inflammatory	Choline salicylate
Azelaic acid	Anti-microbial, anti-inflammatory	Wheat, rye, and barley
Bisabolol	Anti-inflammatory	Chamomile
Borage seed oil	Anti-inflammatory, mild occlusive	Essential fatty acid: gamma-linolenic acid (GLA)
Caper bud extract	Anti-inflammatory	Capparenols
Cucumber extract	Soothing	Cucumber
Evening primrose oil	Anti-inflammatory, mild occlusive	Polyphenols: gallic acid, ellagic acid, pentagalloyl glucose, catechin
Green tea	Anti-inflammatory	Polyphenols: epigallocatechin (EGC) and epigallocatechin-3-gallate (EGCG)
Licorice extract	Soothing	Dipotassium glycyrrhizate
Panthenol	Anti-inflammatory, humectant	Provitamin B5
Sea whip extract	Anti-inflammatory	Coral
Thyme extract	Soothing	Thyme

- **Retinoids** are usually avoided in patients with erythema as the associated retinoid dermatitis tends to be poorly tolerated. Some providers do use non-prescription retinoids in patients with erythema as they are less irritating than prescription-strength retinoids, with the goal to ultimately strengthen the epidermal barrier.

Protect

Physical sunscreens such as zinc oxide and titanium dioxide are preferable in patients with erythema. Chemical sunscreens may release heat when exposed to UV light that can exacerbate erythema. Zinc oxide also has the advantage of functioning as an anti-inflammatory agent. **Antioxidant** products typically contain lower concentrations of key ingredients (e.g., L-ascorbic acid 10%) to reduce potential irritation.

Results

Figure 9 shows a patient with rosacea type I before (A) and after (B) twice daily use for 2 months of a product to reduce inflammation and promote healthy vascular function (containing algae extracts, caperbud and bisabolol), a panthenol-based moisturizer (containing borage and evening primrose oils and aloe vera), and broad-spectrum sunscreen of SPF 30.

Figure 10 shows a patient with facial erythema before (A) and after (B) daily use for 1 week of a glycerin-based moisturizer with licorice, aloe vera and sea whip extract, and a broad-spectrum sunscreen of SPF 30.

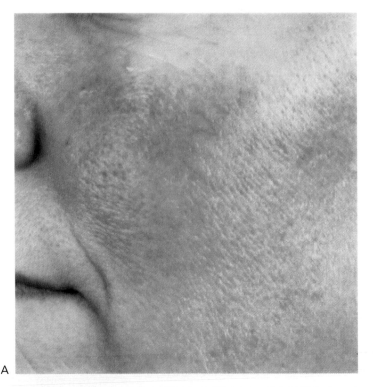

A

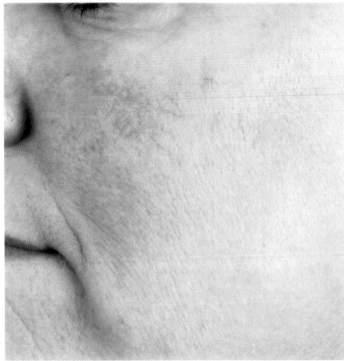

B

FIGURE 9 ● Rosacea type I before **(A)** and after **(B)** daily use for 2 months of a soothing product containing algae extracts, caperbud and bisabolol (Anti-Redness Serum), a panthenol-based lotion moisturizer with borage and evening primrose oils and aloe vera (ReBalance), and a broad-spectrum sunscreen of SPF 30. (Courtesy of PCA SKIN)

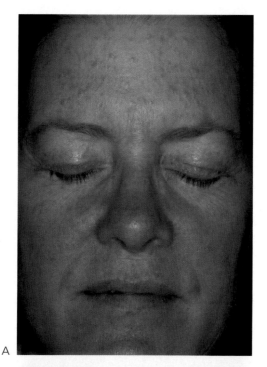

A

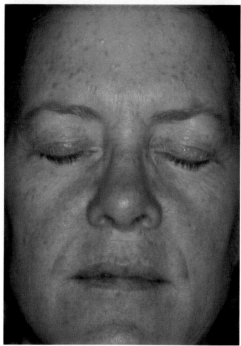

B

FIGURE 10 ● Rosacea type I before **(A)** and after **(B)** daily use for 1 week of glycerin, licorice, aloe vera, lavender, sea whip extract moisturizer, and a broad-spectrum sunscreen of SPF 30 (Obagi Rosaclear System). (Courtesy of Obagi)

Common Follow-ups and Management

During the initial stages of implementing the Topical Product Regimen for Facial Erythema, it is advisable to have the patient return in 4–6 weeks to evaluate the skin, assess tolerability and adherence, and make any necessary adjustments to the regimen. Providers may also inquire about skin dryness and, although unlikely, complications (see Topical Product Complications and Management above).

- **Excessive dryness.** If skin is too dry, an additional hydrating product may be integrated into the regimen such as a hydrating serum (e.g., SkinCeutical's hydrating B5 gel that contains hyaluronic acid and vitamin B5 or PCA SKIN's Hydrating Serum that contains urea, sodium hyaluronate, niacinamide, and glycerin). This may be applied twice daily.
- **Subsequent follow-ups** once patients are satisfied with their topical product regimen are typically every 6 months or as needed to replenish products.

Enhancing Results for Rosacea and Sensitive Skin

Exfoliation procedures such as microdermabrasion and chemical peels for patients with erythematous skin conditions are controversial. The skin barrier is less intact with these conditions relative to normal skin and these exfoliation procedures can regenerate a healthier skin barrier; however, they have the potential to exacerbate erythema and irritation. Lasers and intense pulsed light are very effective at reducing telangiectasias and erythema. Concealing mineral makeup is an option to mask erythema.

Treatment of Acne

Treatment of acne is guided by the presenting lesion types and overall severity. Therapies for noninflammatory acne (acne simplex) focus on exfoliation and reduction of sebum production. Treatment for inflammatory acne (acne vulgaris) includes antibacterials against Propionibacterium acnes (P. acnes) and anti-inflammatory products, in addition to therapies for noninflammatory acne. Moderate to severe cases with numerous papules and pustules warrant oral antibiotics and, for the most severe cases, oral isotretinoin is used.

One possible regimen for treatment of acne (grades I–III) is given below in the Topical Product Regimen for Acne. Many other regimens are possible and equally appropriate. Topical products are often used in conjunction with office-based chemical peels and microdermabrasion exfoliation treatments to maximize results.

Although acne is a condition of excess sebum production, some patients have dehydrated skin due to lack of water content, while others are oily. These different skin types (dehydrated and oily) can help guide the choice of formulation for topical acne products. In general, gels are preferable for oily skin while creams are more hydrating and are preferable for dry skin. In addition, overly aggressive treatment of acne can cause barrier disruption, resulting in dehydration, and increased sebum production perpetuating acne.

● Topical Product Regimen for Acne

Steps	Purpose	Product Type	Example Products with Key Ingredients (Brand Name and Manufacturer)
Cleanse	Remove surface debris and sebum	Medicated cleanser	For example, AHA blend containing glycolic and lactic acid with chamomile and aloe vera (Simply Clean by SkinCeuticals) or salicylic acid 2% (CLENZIderm M.D. Daily Care Foaming Cleanser by Obagi)
Treat	Regulate cellular turnover	Salicylic acid and/or retinoid	For example, Salicylic acid 1.5% with LHA 0.3%, glycolic acid 3.5%, citric acid 0.5% and dioic acid 2% (Blemish and Age Defense by SkinCeuticals) or Retinol 1% (by SkinCeuticals)
	Antibacterial agents (for inflammatory lesions)	Spot treatment	For example, BPO 5% with gluconolactone (Acne Cream by PCA SKIN) or sulfur 10% with salicylic acid (Bye-bye Blemish Drying Lotion by Bye-bye Blemish)
	Maintain hydration levels and anti-inflammatory	Gel, serum or lotion moisturizers	For example, Hyaluronic acid–based gel with thyme and cucumber extracts (Phyto Corrective Gel by SkinCeuticals) or panthenol with borage seed and evening primrose oils, and aloe vera (ReBalance by PCA SKIN)
Protect	Prevent cellular oxidation	Antioxidant	For example, L-ascorbic acid 10% with ferulic acid 0.5% and phloretin 2% serum (Phloretin CF by SkinCeuticals) or L-ascorbic acid 10% (Professional-C Serum by Obagi)
	Prevent damage from UV radiation	Sunscreen	For example, Titanium dioxide 7.3% with zinc oxide 3.4% (Daily Physical Defense SPF 30, SkinMedica) or titanium dioxide 6% with zinc oxide 5% (Sheer Physical UV Defense SPF 50 by SkinCeuticals)

A limited number of products are listed as examples and many other products are equally appropriate.
Indicated for patients with normal to oily skin.

Cleanse

Acne cleansers are designed to reduce sebum and typically foam, due to higher surfactant concentrations. They usually contain active ingredients to further reduce sebum, promote exfoliation, and control bacteria such as benzoyl peroxide (BPO), AHAs, salicylic acid, and sulfur. Abrasives such as scrubs with exfoliating beads and coarse sponges are avoided to prevent excessive irritation and abrasion of fragile skin.

TABLE 4

Acne Therapies

Product	Mechanism of Action
Topical	
Benzoyl peroxide	Antibacterial, anticomedogenic, dessicates skin
Clindamycin	Antibacterial
Erythromycin	Antibacterial
Sodium sulfacetamide	Antibacterial
Retinoids	Exfoliant, comedolytic, and anticomedogenic
Salicylic acid	Exfoliant, comedolytic, anticomedogenic, anti-inflammatory
Dioic oxide	Antibacterial, anticomedogenic
Sulfur	Exfoliant, comedolytic, desiccates skin
Thyme	Antibacterial and anti-inflammatory
Oral	
Isotretinoin	Reduces sebaceous glands and sebum production
Oral contraceptives	Suppresses sebum production by decreasing testosterone
Tetracyclines (tetracycline, minocycline, doxycycline); cephalexin (Keflex); and sulfamethoxazole trimethoprim (Bactrim)	Antibacterial

Treat

Almost all topical acne regimens incorporate exfoliants, anti-inflammatory products, and for papules or pustules, anti-bacterial agents. Table 4 lists commonly used therapies for acne. Many products are labeled as "noncomedogenic"; however, this is not an FDA recognized term nor is there any standardization. "Noncomedogenic" products may be comedogenic or acne causing.

- **Exfoliants** help to regulate follicular keratinization in acne patients. They prevent and treat follicular plugging (commonly referred to as clogged pores), thereby reducing bacteria proliferation and inflammation. Salicylic acid is the most commonly used exfoliant in the treatment of acne. It is **comedolytic** due to its lipophilic properties which allow penetration into sebum-filled pores where it loosens and removes comedonal plugs. Salicylic acid is also **anticomedogenic**, as it prevents follicular plugging and comedone formation, and has anti-inflammatory properties. AHAs such as glycolic and lactic acids may also be used, but they are water-soluble, and as such, are less potent comedolytic agents. Polyhydroxy acids are less irritating than other AHAs, and are commonly used for treatment of acne in patients with sensitive skin. See Treatment of Photoaged Skin above for additional information on exfoliants.
- **Retinoids** reduce acne as well as postinflammatory hyperpigmentation (PIH) which can be associated with acne. Topical retinoid doses are titrated slowly to minimize the associated retinoid dermatitis (see Retinoids section above for information on retinoid dosing). Exacerbation of acne is common during the first few weeks of retinoid use, particularly with prescription retinoids. Retinol and retinaldehyde are less potent alternatives and do not typically cause irritation or increased acne outbreaks.
- **Antibacterial agents** include traditional antibiotics such as topical clindamycin and sodium sulfacetamide and oral tetracyclines, cephalexin and sulfamethoxazole/

trimethoprim. Some cosmeceuticals also have antibacterial activity such as benzoyl peroxide, azelaic acid and kojic acid, but are less potent than prescription products.

- **Benzoyl peroxide (BPO)** has been a standard acne treatment for many years. Its antibacterial activity is due to its ability to release molecular oxygen deep into the hair follicle. Propionibacterium acnes is anaerobic, and through creating this unfavorable environment, BPO rapidly and effectively targets bacteria. BPO also treats acne by decreasing bacterial resistance to systemic and topical antibiotics, and it functions as an exfoliant. BPO products cause dryness and can be associated with skin irritation. Providers are encouraged to use lower concentrations of 2.5% on the full face, as these are associated with less irritation and equivalent efficacy to products with higher percentages of BPO. Spot treatments and cleansers, which are either applied to small areas or for short periods of time, typically have higher percentages of BPO such as 5%.
- **Azelaic acid** is a multifunctional product that can be used to treat acne, rosacea, and hyperpigmentation. Its anti-acne benefits are attributed to its keratolytic, antibacterial, and anti-inflammatory properties. In addition, it is not affected by bacterial resistance. Prescription azelaic acid products contain up to 20%, while cosmeceutical products typically contain up to 5% azelaic acid. All strengths have been shown to be beneficial for acne.
- **Kojic acid** is typically used for prevention and treatment of hyperpigmentation. It also has antibacterial activity and so is a useful therapy for acne and PIH.
- **Dioic acid** is derived from oleic acid. It is and is used for treatment of hyperpigmentation and acne, as it inhibits sebum production and has antibacterial activity against P. acnes.
- **Anti-inflammatory agents** (Table 3) are also used to treat inflammatory acne and are listed in Table 3, Cosmeceuticals for Facial Erythema.
- **Astringent agents** such as ginger root extract and witch hazel help control excessive sebum production. Disposable pads saturated with these products may be used as needed, no more than twice daily, if oiliness persists after consistent use of the Topical Product Regimen. These are particularly useful in adolescent patients who have hormonally induced sebum production.

Protect

Sunscreen use in patients with acne is important as some anti-acne products can increase photosensitivity, such as tetracycline, doxycycline, retinoids and BPO. Erythema associated with inflammatory lesions, particularly in unprotected skin, can lead to PIH. Patients with acne are often wary of sunscreens as thick sunscreen creams can contribute to acne formation. Therefore, broad-spectrum sunscreens with SPF 30 or greater are recommended in thin lotion formulations. **Antioxidants** are also recommended to help reduce harmful oxidative effects of UV exposure.

Results

Figure 11 shows a patient with severe acne vulgaris before (A) and after (B) daily use for 2 months of an alpha hydroxy acid cleanser, tretinoin gel 0.05%, hyaluronic acid gel moisturizer with cucumber and thyme, and a broad-spectrum sunscreen of SPF 30.

Figure 12 shows a patient with mild to moderate acne vulgaris before (A) and after (B) daily use for 2 months of an alpha hydroxy acid cleanser, retinol 0.5%, salicylic acid 2%, azelaic acid 5% spot treatment, lotion moisturizer, and a broad-spectrum sunscreen of SPF 30.

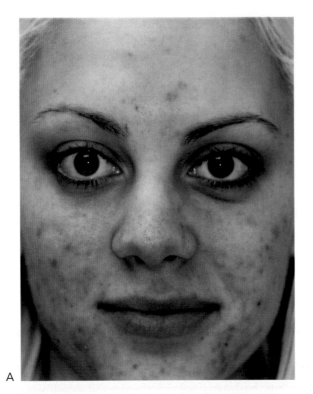

A

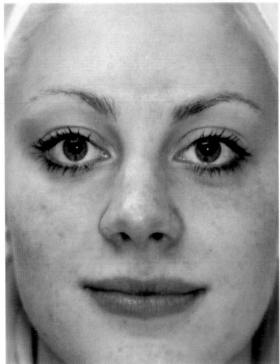

B

FIGURE 11 ● Acne vulgaris before **(A)** and after **(B)** daily use for 2 months of an alpha hydroxy acid cleanser (Simply Clean), tretinoin gel 0.05% (Atralin), soothing hyaluronic acid base gel moisturizer with cucumber and thyme (Phyto Corrective Gel), and a broad-spectrum sunscreen of SPF 30 (Daily Physical Defense). (Courtesy of Rebecca Small, MD)

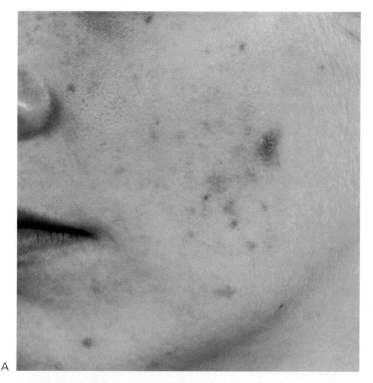

A

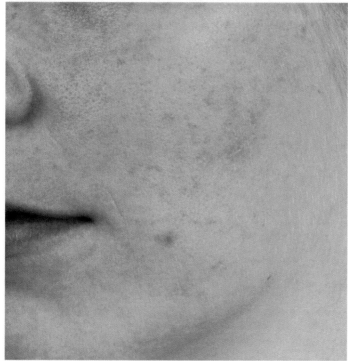

B

FIGURE 12 ● Acne vulgaris before **(A)** and after **(B)** daily use for 2 months of an alpha hydroxy acid cleanser, retinol 0.5% (A&C Synergy Serum), salicylic acid 2% and azelaic acid 5% spot treatment (Acne Gel), soothing moisturizer lotion with aloe vera, allantoin, bisabolol, borage seed oil (Clearskin) and a broad-spectrum sunscreen of SPF 30. (Courtesy of PCA SKIN)

Figure 13 shows a patient with mild to moderate acne vulgaris before (A) and after (B) daily use for 2 weeks of a salicylic acid cleanser, salicylic acid 2% serum, glycerin 20% lotion moisturizer, and a broad-spectrum sunscreen of SPF 30.

Common Follow-ups and Management

During the initial stages of implementing a Topical Product Regimen for Acne, it is advisable to have the patient return in 4–6 weeks to evaluate the skin, assess tolerability and adherence, and to make any necessary adjustments to their regimen. Patients are also evaluated for skin dryness, oiliness, irritation, and although unlikely, complications (see below).

- **Excessive dryness.** If skin is too dry, an additional hydrating product may be integrated into the regimen such as a hydrating serum (e.g., SkinCeutical's Hydrating B5 Gel which contains hyaluronic acid and vitamin B5, or PCA SKIN's Hydrating Serum that contains urea, sodium hyaluronate, niacinamide, and glycerin).
- **Excessive oiliness.** Salicylic acid infused pads (e.g., NeoStrata's NeoCeuticals Acne Treatment Solution Pads) may be used to wipe the skin especially on the forehead, nose, and chin ("T-zone") during the day if oily. This should be followed by a reapplication of a broad-spectrum sunscreen of SPF 30 or greater appropriate for acne.
- **Excessive irritation.** If skin is too irritated, consider adding a soothing product that contains anti-inflammatory ingredients (e.g., PCA SKIN's Anti-Redness Serum that contains dimethicone and algae extracts, or SkinCeutical's Phyto Corrective Gel that contains hyaluronic acid, thyme, and cucumber).
- **Subsequent follow-ups** once patients are satisfied with their skin care regimen are typically every 6 months or as needed to replenish products.

Enhancing Results for Acne

Combining topical products with **exfoliation procedures** such as chemical peels and microdermabrasion can enhance results for both noninflammatory and inflammatory acne. A series of superficial chemical peels (e.g., salicylic acid or Jessner's peels) and/or microdermabrasion enhances exfoliation and reduces follicular plugging and inflammation. Exfoliation also accelerates pigment removal and can reduce PIH. Chemical peels and microdermabrasion are readily performed in patients using nonprescription retinoids; however, integration with prescription retinoids is more challenging (see Retinoids above).

    Light-based therapies are treatment options for inflammatory acne. The mechanism of action of light-based treatments hinges on the fact that the P. acnes produces porphyrins. When bacterial porphyrins are exposed to light, particularly blue light (415 nm), free radicals are produced and a cytotoxic reaction ensues which selectively kills the bacteria. Although red light (635 nm) is less effective at porphyrin photoactivation, it penetrates deeper into the skin and light-based treatments for acne, therefore, often combine both red and blue light. **Photodynamic therapy** employs the use of topical photosensitizing medications such as aminolevulinic acid (Levulan) to selectively destroy targeted tissues. Aminolevulinic acid is concentrated in P. acnes and sebaceous glands, and upon activation with a light source such as intense pulsed light, red or blue light, or a pulsed dye laser (595 nm), a localized cytotoxic reaction occurs resulting in destruction of these targets.

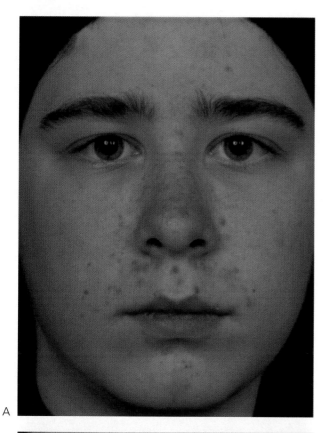

A

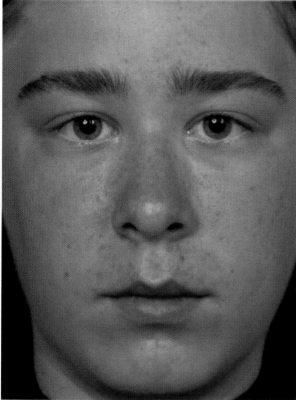

B

FIGURE 13 ● Acne vulgaris before **(A)** and after **(B)** daily use for 2 weeks of a salicylic acid cleanser, salicylic acid 2% serum, glycerin 20% lotion moisturizer, and a broad-spectrum sunscreen of SPF 30 (CLENZIderm MD, Obagi). (Courtesy of Obagi)

Treatment of Hyperpigmentation

Treatment of hyperpigmentation with topical products is aimed at suppressing melanin synthesis (melanogenesis) and removing pigment that is already present in the skin through exfoliation (Fig. 14). In addition, products associated with irritation are avoided, particularly in dark Fitzpatrick skin types (IV–VI), as prolonged irritation can stimulate melanogenesis.

This section focuses on a targeted group of topical skin care products used for treatment and prevention of hyperpigmentation, referred to as the Topical Product Regimen for Hyperpigmentation (see below). Many alternative selections of topical products are equally appropriate. This regimen is typically utilized in conjunction with in-office superficial chemical peels and microdermabrasion exfoliation treatments to enhance results.

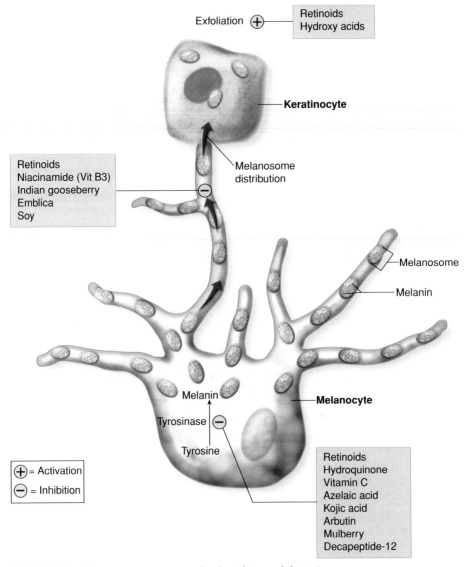

FIGURE 14 ● Hyperpigmentation pathophysiology and therapies.

● Topical Product Regimen for Hyperpigmentation

Steps	Purpose	Product Type	Example Products with Key Ingredients (Brand Name and Manufacturer)
Cleanse	Remove surface debris, sebum	Gentle facial cleanser	For example, Cream cleanser (Creamy Cleanser by PCA SKIN or Gentle Cleanser by SkinCeuticals)
Treat	Inhibit melanogenesis	Tyrosinase inhibitor	For example, Hydroquinone 4% (Clear by Obagi) or hydroquinone 2% with kojic acid (Pigment Gel by PCA SKIN) or kojic acid 2% with emblica 2% and glycolic acid (Pigment Regulator by SkinCeuticals)
	Regulate cellular turnover	Retinoid	For example, Retinol 1% (by SkinCeuticals), or retinol 1% with retinyl palmitate 0.1% and retinyl acetate 0.1% (Tri-retinol Complex by SkinMedica)
	Maintain hydration levels	Moisturizer	For example, Panthenol and mango butter-based cream with oils of grape seed, rose hip, and macademia (Emollience by SkinCeuticals) or petrolatum-based cream with dimethicone, sweet almond oil and tocopherol acetate (Cetaphil Cream by Galderma).
Protect	Prevent cellular oxidation	Antioxidant	For example, L-ascorbic acid 15% with alpha tocopherol 1% and ferulic acid (CE Ferulic by SkinCeuticals) or L-ascorbic acid 20% (Professional-C Serum by Obagi)
	Prevent damage from UV adiation	Sunscreen	For example, Titanium dioxide 7.3% with zinc oxide 3.4% (Daily Physical Defense SPF 30 by SkinMedica) or zinc oxide 7% with octinoxate 7.5% (Ultimate UV Defense SPF 30 by SkinCeuticals)

A limited number of products are listed as examples and many other products are equally appropriate. Indicated for patients with normal to dry skin.

Cleanse

Patients with hyperpigmentation can have a variety of skin types. A cream-based cleanser is recommended for normal to dry skin and a foaming cleanser for oily skin types.

Treat

Inhibition of melanin synthesis is one of the most important functions of topical products used in the treatment of hyperpigmentation. Conversion of tyrosine to melanin by tyrosinase is the key step in melanogenesis, and tyrosinase inhibitors are the primary topical lightening agents used for hyperpigmentation (Fig. 14). Topical lightening agents are available as prescription products that have potent active ingredients at higher concentrations (Table 5). Topical brightening agents are also available as cosmeceutical products (Table 6). "Lightening" is an FDA-regulated term and is applied to prescription medications such as hydroquinone; whereas, "brightening" is used to describe cosmeceutical products.

- **Hydroquinone** is one of the most potent melanogenesis inhibitors. It suppresses melanin synthesis by inhibiting tyrosinase, decreases melanosome formation, increases melanosome degradation, and induces melanocyte-specific cytotoxicity. It is available

TABLE 5

Prescription Topical Products for Treatment of Hyperpigmentation

Product Trade Name	Lightening Ingredient	Retinoid	Sun Protectant	Other Components
Finacea	Azelaic acid 15%	None	None	
Claripel	HQ 4%	None	Sunscreen	
Eldopaque Forte	HQ 4%	None	Sunscreen	
Eldoquin Forte	HQ 4%	None	None	
EpiQuin	HQ 4%	Retinol 0.15%		Vitamins C and E
Glyquin	HQ 4%	None	Sunscreen	Vitamins C and E Glycolic acid 10%
Glyquin XM	HQ 4%	None	Sunscreen	Vitamins C and E Hyaluronic acid
Lustra	HQ 4%	None		Vitamins C and E Glycolic acid 2%
Lustra AF	HQ 4%	None	Sunscreen	Vitamins C and E Glycolic acid 2%
Lustra Ultra	HQ 4%	None	Sunscreen	Petrolatum
Alustra	HQ 4%	Retinol	None	
Melquin	HQ 4%	None	None	Petrolatum
Nuquin	HQ 4%	None	Sunscreen	Petrolatum
Obagi Nu-Derm Clear	HQ 4%	None	None	Vitamins C and E Lactic acid
Obagi-C Night Therapy	HQ 4%	None	None	Vitamins C and E Lactic acid Salicylic acid
Solage	Mequinol 2%	Retinoic acid 0.01%	None	
Solaquin Forte	HQ 4%	None	Sunscreen	
Triluma	HQ 4%	Retinoic acid 0.05%		Fluocinolone acetonide 0.01%

HQ = Hydroquinone.

as an OTC drug in 2% formulations and can be prescribed in 4% creams or formulated up to 8% by compounding pharmacies. Hydroquinone can cause irritation. Gradually increasing the frequency of use from every other evening to nightly over 2 weeks can reduce the likelihood of irritation. Because of its cytotoxic effect on melanocytes, hydroquinone has been prohibited for use in certain countries abroad. For this reason, many manufacturers in the United States have developed other cosmeceutical lightening agents as alternatives to hydroquinone.

- **Cosmeceuticals** also have skin brightening properties. Some function as tyrosinase inhibitors such as kojic acid and arbutin; however, they are not as effective as hydroquinone. Of the cosmeceutical agents available, azelaic acid, kojic acid, and arbutin are some of the most potent. Kojic acid has potential for irritation and has been associated with irritant dermatitis.

TABLE 6

Cosmeceutical Topical Products for Treatment of Hyperpigmentation

Ingredient	Source
Acetyl glucosamine	Chitin
Aloesin	Aloe vera
Arbutin	Bearberry
Azelaic acid	Pityrosporum ovale derivative
Dioic acid	Oleic acid derivative
Emblica	Indian gooseberry
Glycolic acid	Sugarcane
Hydroquinone	Synthetic
Kojic acid	Fungi
Licorice extract (glabridin)	Licorice root
Lumixyl (peptide)	Decapeptide-12
Mulberry extract	Broussonetia papyrifera tree root
Niacinamide	Vitamin B3 amide
Phenylethyl resorcinol	Resorcinol derivative (synthetic)
Retinoids	Vitamin A derivatives
Soy flavonoids	Soybean
Undecylenoyl phenylalanine	Synthetic melanocyte stimulating hormone (MSH) suppressor
Vitamin C	Citrus fruits

- **Retinoids** inhibit tyrosinase activity, melanosome distribution, and promote exfoliation. Prescription retinoids have the most profound effect on reducing hyperpigmentation. However, they can be poorly tolerated due to the retinoid dermatitis associated with their use. Nonprescription retinoids such as retinol are less potent alternatives and are rarely associated with irritation.
- **Combining lightening agents** with exfoliants such as AHAs or retinoids, enhances penetration into the skin and renders products more effective than when used individually. The classic compounded triple cream, Tri-Luma, is an FDA-approved product for the treatment of melasma which contains hydroquinone 4%, tretinoin 0.05% and a corticosteroid (fluocinolone acetonide 0.01%). Steroids may be added to prescription retinoid products to reduce irritation; however, caution is advised with these as chronic use can thin the skin and stimulate telangiectasia formation. Mequinol, a synthetic hydroquinone derivative, is available as a combination product of mequinol 2% with tretinoin 0.01% (Solage). Cosmeceutical brightening agents are also commonly combined to maximize penetration and efficacy, such as kojic acid with retinol or glycolic acid (e.g., SkinCeutical's Pigment Regulator contains kojic acid 2%, emblica 2%, and glycolic acid or PCA SKIN's Intensive Clarity Treatment with 0.5% retinol, lactic acid and gluconolactone.)
- **Growth factors** may be used in patients with hyperpigmentation and are often incorporated after the initial topical product regimen is well established. While growth factor products are primarily used for collagen stimulation to reduce wrinkles, some products such as NouriCel-MD (by SkinMedica) also clinically demonstrate reduction of hyperpigmentation.

Protect

Diligent sun protective measures with daily use of a broad-spectrum **sunscreen** of SPF 30 or greater containing zinc oxide or titanium dioxide are an essential part of treatment in all patients with hyperpigmentation. A topical **antioxidant**, such as L-ascorbic acid, is also used daily in the morning for UV protection and for its skin lightening properties. In addition, because melanin is a natural defense mechanism against the sun, reducing the amount of pigment in the skin has some theoretical risks and use of these protective products helps mitigate these risks.

Results

Figure 15 shows a patient with PIH secondary to acne before (A) and after (B) daily use for 3 months of retinol 0.5%, hydroquinone 2%, kojic acid, azelaic acid, resorcinol, arbutin, undecylenoyl phenylalanine, and a broad-spectrum sunscreen of SPF 30.

Figure 16 shows a patient with PIH secondary to a chemical peel before (A) and after (B) daily use for 4 months of hydroquinone 2%, kojic acid, azelaic acid, and a broad-spectrum sunscreen of SPF 30.

Figure 17 shows a patient with melasma before (A) and after (B) twice daily use for 2 months of hydroquinone 4%, and daily use of 0.1% retinoic acid, glycolic acid 6% with lactic acid 4%, and a broad-spectrum sunscreen of SPF 30.

Common Follow-ups and Management

During the initial stages of implementing a Topical Product Regimen for Hyperpigmentation, it is advisable to have the patient return in 4–6 weeks to evaluate the skin, assess tolerability and adherence, and to make any necessary adjustments to their regimen. Patients are also evaluated for skin irritation and, although unlikely, complications (see below).

- **Irritation.** Hydroquinone and retinoids can cause irritation. Reducing the dose by cutting the quantity applied in half, or reducing the frequency of use from daily to every other day, can often alleviate irritation. If skin irritation persists, consider switching to an alternative non-hydroquinone, non-retinoid product (e.g., SkinCeutical's Pigment Regulator containing kojic acid 2% with emblica 2% and glycolic acid).
- **Subsequent follow-ups** once patients are satisfied with their skin care regimen are typically every 6 months or as needed to replenish products.

Enhancing Results for Hyperpigmentation

Exfoliation procedures such as chemical peels and microdermabrasion are often used in combination with topical products to accelerate and enhance results. Combining **lasers and light-based procedures** which target unwanted pigment with exfoliation treatments and topical products achieves the most profound reduction in UV-induced and postinflammatory hyperpigmentation. Discontinuation of **exogenous hormones** such as oral contraceptives is recommended when possible in patients with melasma. Avoiding aggressive aesthetic procedures in patients with dark Fitzpatrick skin types (IV–VI) is also helpful in preventing procedure-related PIH.

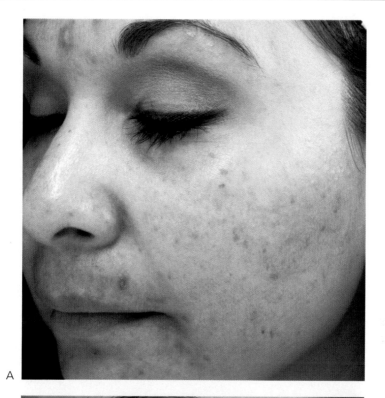

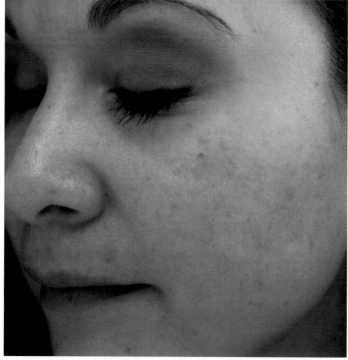

FIGURE 15 ● Postinflammatory hyperpigmentation secondary to acne before **(A)** and after **(B)** daily use for 3 months of retinol 0.5% (A&C Synergy Serum), hydroquinone 2% with kojic acid, azelaic acid and lactic acid (Pigment Gel), resorcinol, arbutin, and undecylenoyl phenylalanine (Brightening Therapy with True Tone), and a broad-spectrum sunscreen of SPF 30. (Courtesy of PCA SKIN)

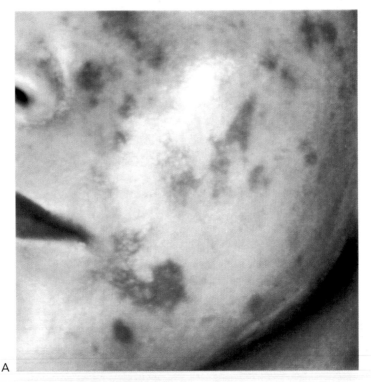

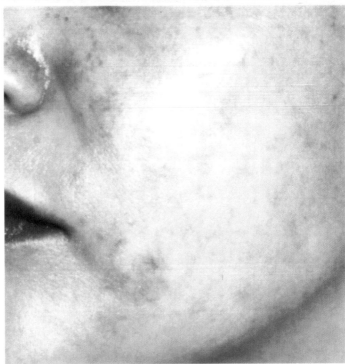

FIGURE 16 ● Postinflammatory hyperpigmentation secondary to a chemical peel before **(A)** and after **(B)** daily use for 4 months of hydroquinone 2% with kojic acid, azelaic acid and lactic acid (Pigment Gel), and a broad-spectrum sunscreen of SPF 30. (Courtesy of PCA SKIN)

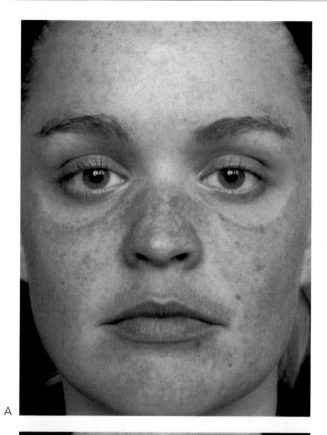

A

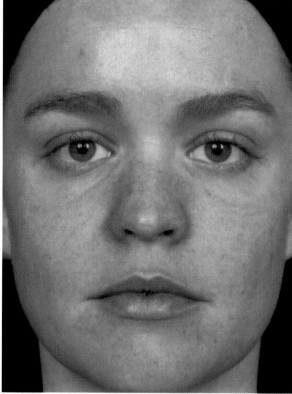

B

FIGURE 17 ● Melasma before **(A)** and after **(B)** use for 2 months of twice daily hydroquinone 4%, and daily 0.1% retinoic acid, glycolic acid 6% with lactic acid 4%, and a broad-spectrum sunscreen of SPF 30 (Nu-Derm System). (Courtesy of Obagi)

Skin Care Products for Pre and Postprocedure

Topical skin care products are used before and after aesthetic procedures, such as chemical peels and laser treatments, to support and enhance results. They prepare skin by creating a healthier baseline epidermis and dermis prior to procedures, and they soothe skin and promote healing postprocedure. Use of lightening agents can also reduce the risk of pigmentary complications after procedures such as PIH.

Preprocedure

Topical skin care products for preprocedure use typically consist of a retinoid, moisturizer, antioxidant, sunscreen, and may include a growth factor, which are the same products used in the Topical Product Regimen for Photoaged Skin. A topical lightening agent, such as hydroquinone 2–8%, may also be added to help reduce the risk of postprocedure PIH in patients prone to hyperpigmentation, such as dark Fitzpatrick skin types (IV–VI). Use of a preprocedure topical product regimen 1–2 months prior to aesthetic procedures conditions the skin by thinning the stratum corneum and stimulates epidermal renewal. This allows for more even penetration of products during treatment such as chemical peels and facilitates healing. To ensure that the epidermis is fully intact at the time of treatment, prescription retinoids are discontinued 1–2 weeks prior to procedure, and hydroxy acids are discontinued 1 week prior to procedure.

Postprocedure

Selection of postprocedure products is determined by the type of cosmetic procedure performed and whether the skin is intact or nonintact after completion of the procedure.

Treatments which leave the epidermis intact, such as nonablative lasers and superficial resurfacing treatments like chemical peels and microdermabrasion, are managed postprocedure with **nonocclusive** topical products. These nonocclusive products contain active ingredients to soothe skin (such as borage and evening primrose seed oils) and promote healing (such as beta glucan and peptides). Table 7 lists commonly used nonocclusive postprocedure products. A gentle cleanser and broad-spectrum sunscreen of SPF 30 or greater containing zinc oxide or titanium dioxide are used in addition to the nonocclusive product for 1–2 weeks postprocedure. Patients may resume their routine topical regimen, such as the Topical Product Regimen for Photoaged Skin, 1–2 weeks postprocedure when the skin is no longer erythematous.

TABLE 7

Nonocclusive Postprocedure Products

Product Brand Name (Manufacturer)	Ingredients (Intended Effect or Product Type)
Biafine (OrthoNeutrogena)	Trolamin salicylate, sodium alginate (wound healing)
Epidermal Repair (SkinCeuticals)	Beta glucan and Centella asiatica (collagen synthesis)
ReBalance (PCA SKIN)	Borage seed oil and evening primrose seed oil (anti-inflammatory), panthenol and niacinamide (moisturizers), and tocopherol (antioxidant)
TNS Ceramide Treatment Cream (SkinMedica)	Hydroxypropyl bispalmitamide MEA (ceramide for barrier enhancement), NouriCel-MD (growth factors), palmitoyl oligopeptide and palmitoyl tetrapeptide-7 (matrix synthesis)

TABLE 8

Occlusive Postprocedure Products

Product Brand Name (Manufacturer)	Hydrating Ingredients	Other Ingredients
Aquaphor (Beiersdorf)	Mineral oil Lanolin	Panthenol Bisapolol
Catrix 10 (Lescarden)	Petrolatum Beeswax Paraffin	Bovine mucopolysaccharide cartilage 10%
Primacy (SkinCeuticals)	Petrolatum Squalene Oat kernel oil Rose oil	Bisabolol Aloe vera Vitamin E
Protective Recovery Balm (BiO2 Cosmeceuticals)	Mineral oil Petrolatum Paraffin Dimethicone	
Puralube (Nycomed)	Light mineral oil White petrolatum	

   Treatments which ablate the epidermis, such as laser resurfacing, deeper chemical peels, and dermabrasion are managed immediately postprocedure with an occlusive moisturizer that facilitates re-epithelialization through moist wound healing. These **occlusive** products are usually formulated as ointments and primarily contain ingredients for intense hydration. Some also contain active ingredients to soothe skin and promote healing. Common occlusive postprocedure products are shown in Table 8. Puralube is an ophthalmologic grade petrolatum product which may be used in the periocular area. Occlusive postprocedure products may be applied immediately after completion of the procedure and continued until re-epithelialization occurs. This is usually for 4–7 days after fractional ablative lasers, and up to 2 weeks or more after nonfractional ablative lasers, medium and deep chemical peels, and dermabrasion. The skin may be cleansed with dilute acetic acid (gauze soaked in a solution of 1 tsp of white vinegar in 2 cups of water) up to 4 times per day to reduce the risk of infection. As most of these products are ointments, it is not possible to layer other products such as sunscreen on top of them. Therefore, sun protective measures such as hats and sun avoidance during this period of healing are very important. Prolonged use of occlusive products can be associated with acne and milia (see Topical Product Complications and Management above).

   Once the skin has fully re-epithelialized, a nonocclusive product (Table 7) may be used along with a gentle cleanser and a daily broad-spectrum sunscreen of SPF 30 or greater containing zinc oxide or titanium dioxide. Patients may resume their routine topical regimen, such as the Topical Product Regimen for Photoaged Skin, approximately 1 month postprocedure when the skin is no longer erythematous or sensitive. If PIH is a concern, skin lightening products may also be started 1 month postprocedure.

Skin Structure and Function

Skin Function

Overall	The skin is the largest organ of the body and serves as an elastic protective covering that provides antimicrobial, chemoprotective, and physical barrier functions.
Heat regulation	The skin regulates body temperature through production and evaporation of perspiration for cooling. The sudoriferous glands are responsible for perspiration. These glands include the eccrine and apocrine glands and are found throughout cutaneous (epidermis and dermis) and subcutaneous tissues. Perspiration is composed of water, fatty acids, and minerals.
Absorption	The permeability of the skin is regulated by the acid mantle layer of the epidermis. It is comprised of perspiration, sebum, keratin, lactic acid, urea, and other substances found in the epidermis. The low pH provides antibacterial and antifungal benefits, and limits the amount of external substances capable of entering and affecting the body.
Secretion	Sebaceous glands excrete sebum, or oil, to lubricate the skin. Sebum is made up of squalene, cholesterol, triglycerides, and other lipids, all of which are important for skin protection and moisturization.
Protection	Subcutaneous adipose tissue provides insulation and protection against trauma to the internal organs. The skin has other protective functions as a microbial barrier and offers protection from the harmful effects of ultraviolet (UV) radiation through the production of melanin. Through absorbing UV radiation, melanin reduces the penetration of UV rays into the skin and protects keratinocyte nuclei against its mutagenic effects.
Excretion	Perspiration eliminates waste materials through sudoriferous gland excretion and regulates body temperature.
Sensation	Nerve fibers span the dermal layer and perceive heat, cold, touch, pleasure, pressure, and pain.

Skin Structure

Overall	The different layers of the skin contain numerous components responsible for overall healthy skin function (see Anatomy section, Fig. 1).
Epidermis	The epidermis typically consists of 5–6 separate layers (depending on the body location) (see Anatomy section, Fig. 3). As the outermost portion of the skin, the epidermis plays a vital protective role against external factors that necessitates constant renewal.
Stratum corneum (cornified layer)	This epidermal layer contains tightly packed non-viable cells (corneocytes) that are constantly shed and replaced. Keratinocytes produced in the stratum basale of the epidermis migrate up through the epidermis until they complete their life cycle by transforming into flattened corneocytes that integrate into the stratum corneum. Corneocytes are shed from the skin surface (see Anatomy section, Fig. 3). This entire process is known as the epidermal maturation process or cellular turnover and takes an estimated 28 days. The stratum corneum contains the skin's natural moisturizing factor (NMF), which is responsible for maintaining hydration within the stratum corneum. NMF exists inside the corneocytes and consists of urea, magnesium, ammonia, phosphate, uric acid, chlorine, amino acids, citrate, sodium PCA, sodium potassium, lactate, calcium, glucosamine, sugar, peptides, organic acids, and other unidentified substances. Surrounding the corneocytes is the lipid bilayer, which maintains moisture in the stratum corneum. This thin membrane is comprised of 2 layers of phospholipids that have a hydrophilic head and two hydrophobic tails. They naturally arrange themselves with all of their tails pointing toward one another, creating the bilayer. Most hydrating products are designed to replicate NMF and lipids in the stratum corneum, and these naturally occurring components are frequently used in moisturizers.
Stratum lucidum (clear layer)	This epidermal layer contains transparent cells and is only present in areas with the thickest skin on the body, such as the palms of the hands and soles of the feet. Unlike the other layers of the skin, light can pass through the stratum lucidum.
Stratum granulosum (granular layer)	This epidermal layer consists of matured keratinocyte cells. They contain granules that were originally intracellular organelles in their immature basal cell form.
Stratum spinosum (spinous layer)	This epidermal layer contains multiple layers of flattened, square-shaped cells. The desmosomal bonds that hold the spinous layer together have a spiny appearance when viewed under a microscope. The stratum spinosum also contains Langerhans cells, which are part of the immune system and aid in immune surveillance in the skin.
Stratum basale (stratum germinativum)	This epidermal layer consists of immature keratinocytes (which are squamous cells), capable of cell division and are responsible for growth and renewal of the epidermis. All cells of the epidermis start at the stratum basale and migrate through the other layers until they become a part of the stratum corneum and are eventually shed from the skin's surface. Melanocytes, the skin's pigment-producing cells, reside in the basal layer as well.
Dermis	The dermis lies below the epidermis and consists of 2 layers, the papillary and reticular dermis. It is comprised of reticular fibers, vascular structures, and various connective tissues. The dermis provides support and structure for the epidermal layers.
Papillary dermis	The more superficial dermal layer. It has cone-shaped projections, called papillae, that reach into the epidermis and contain blood vessels and nerve fibers, referred to as tactile corpuscles. Papillae are responsible for nourishing the epidermis and tactile corpuscles provide sensation.

Skin Structure (*Continued*)

Reticular dermis	The deepest portion of the dermis. This dermal layer contains the extracellular matrix (ECM), lymph nodes, sebaceous and sudoriferous glands, fibrous and elastic tissue, as well as blood vessels and nerves.
Extracellular matrix	The extracellular matrix surrounds the cells and provides supportive and protective benefits. The ECM consists of structural proteins, glycosaminoglycans, proteoglycans, and adhesive proteins. Matrix metalloproteinase enzymes are also present and work to break down and recycle spent ECM components.

Structural proteins

- Collagen is the predominant protein making up the ECM. There are numerous types of collagen, and types I, III, and IV are commonly found in the skin. New collagen production slows and destruction of collagen speeds up as a result of the natural aging process.
- Elastin is the protein that comprises the core of elastic fibers and allows cutaneous structures to stretch easily without breaking. Elastin is not as widely distributed as collagen in the dermis. Elasticity decreases over time due to calcification and damage of elastin fibers.

Glycosaminoglycans and proteoglycans

Glycosaminoglycans (GAGs) are polysaccharides that reside in the ECM. All bond to matrix proteins to form proteoglycans, with the exception of hyaluronic acid. Glycosaminoglycans include:

- Hyaluronic acid (HA) augments skin thickness by increasing hydration. HA is critical to skin hydration due to its hygroscopic properties, or the ability to attract and bind water in the skin. HA has the capacity to hold up to 1000 times its molecular weight in water moisture.
- Chondroitin sulfate facilitates migration of other molecules through tissues, maintaining nutrient levels and aiding in skin flexibility and strength.
- Heparin sulfate is vital to cellular division and the regulation of other cellular functions.
- Dermatan sulfate contributes to the stability of the dermis and limits cell migration and proliferation.

Adhesive proteins

- Fibronectin and laminins attach cells to the extracellular matrix.

Matrix metalloproteinases

Matrix metalloproteinases (MMPs) are enzymes that are responsible for recycling of matrix proteins. While they are critical for breaking down old, worn-out proteins, unfortunately, MMPs can be overproduced as a result of sun exposure. Excessive MMP activity associated with the unwanted breakdown of healthy proteins can accelerate visible signs of aging. Certain skin care products contain MMP inhibitors that are aimed at preventing and treating skin aging.

- Collagenase breaks down collagen
- Elastase breaks down elastin
- Hyaluronidase breaks down hyaluronic acid

(Continued)

Skin Structure (*Continued*)

Sebaceous glands

These small oil-producing glands secrete sebum into the hair follicles, which eventually reaches the skin's surface. Sebum lubricates and prevents moisture loss from the skin. These glands are found in all parts of the body excluding the palms of the hands and soles of the feet. Androgen hormones are stimulatory factors for these glands. Upregulation by testosterone and dihydrotestosterone increases the size and activity of the sebaceous glands; this is frequently experienced during puberty and with exogenous hormones. Acne-controlling skin care products can be used to help control sebum production.

Sudoriferous glands (sweat glands)

These glands are responsible for temperature regulation and excretion of wastes. Although present in most parts of the body, sudoriferous glands are more predominant on the palms of the hands, soles of the feet, forehead, and underarms. There are two types of sudoriferous glands found in the skin: eccrine and apocrine glands.

- Eccrine glands secrete the watery sweat that is released in response to heat. The eccrine glands' purpose is to keep the body cool through evaporation.

- Apocrine glands are larger and deeper in the skin than eccrine glands, and are associated with the hair follicle. Apocrine glands produce thicker secretions that contain pheromones which emit odors. Apocrine glands do not become active until puberty.

Subcutaneous layer	The subcutaneous layer of the skin lies below the dermis and is made up primarily of adipose (fat) cells. It also contains larger blood vessels, lymph channels, and connective tissue. The thickness of this layer varies from person to person, as well as over different locations of the body. Temperature regulation and protection from injury are important roles of the subcutaneous layer.

Patient Intake Form

Date:_____

NAME:_____ AGE:_____ * DOB:_____
         Last   First

ADDRESS:_____ CITY:_____ ZIP:_____

HOME PHONE:_____ ☐ OK TO CONTACT/LEAVE MESSAGE HERE

MOBILE PHONE:_____ ☐ OK TO CONTACT/LEAVE MESSAGE HERE

WORK PHONE:_____ ☐ OK TO CONTACT/LEAVE MESSAGE HERE

E-MAIL:_____ ☐ OK TO CONTACT/LEAVE MESSAGE HERE

OCCUPATION:_____ REFERRED BY:_____

In order of importance, beginning with 1, make a wish list of what you would like to see improved in your skin in the next 30 days:
_____ Reduction of fine lines _____ Reduction of oil/acne _____ Reduction of redness _____ Reduction of brown spots/sun damage
_____ Reduction of hair _____ Acne scars diminished _____ Tattoo   *For minors, please list guardian info.

Medical history	Yes	No
Are you or is it possible that you may be pregnant?		
Are you breastfeeding?		
Do you form thick or raised scars from cuts or burns?		
After injury to the skin (such as cuts/burns) do you have: (circle) Darkening of the skin in that area (hyperpigmentation) Lightening of the skin in that area (hypopigmentation)		
Hair removal by plucking, waxing, electrolysis in the last 4 weeks?		
Tanning (tanning bed) or sun exposure in the last 4 weeks? (circle)		
Tanning products or spray on tan in the last 2 weeks?		
Do you have a tan now in the area to be treated?		
Do you use sunscreen daily with spf 30 or higher?		
History of skin cancer or unusual moles?		
Have you ever had a photosensitive disorder? (e.g., lupus)		
History of seizures?		
Permanent make-up or tattoos? Where _____		
Have you used Accutane in last 6 months?		
Are you currently taking antibiotics? Which _____		
Are you using Retin-A or glycolic acid products? (circle)		
Are you currently under the care of a physician?		
Do you currently smoke?		
Do you have an allergy or sensitivity to lidocaine, latex, sulfa medications, aspirin, hydroquinone, aloe, bee stings? (circle)		
Life threatening allergy to anything?		
Do you have scars on the face?		

Explanation of items marked "Yes":
_____
_____
_____
_____

Please check all medical conditions past or present	Yes	No
Keloid scarring	☐	☐
Cold sores	☐	☐
Herpes (genital)	☐	☐
Easy bruising or bleeding	☐	☐
Active skin infection	☐	☐
Moles that changed, itched, or bled	☐	☐
Recent increase in amount of hair	☐	☐
Asthma	☐	☐
Seasonal allergies/allergic rhinitis	☐	☐
Eczema	☐	☐
Thyroid imbalance	☐	☐
Poor healing	☐	☐
Diabetes	☐	☐
Heart condition	☐	☐
High blood pressure	☐	☐
Pacemaker	☐	☐
Disease of nerves or muscles (e.g., ALS, myasthenia gravis, Lambert–Eaton or other)	☐	☐
Cancer	☐	☐
HIV/AIDS	☐	☐
Autoimmune disease (e.g., rheumatoid arthritis, scleroderma)	☐	☐
Hepatitis	☐	☐
Shingles	☐	☐
Migraine headaches	☐	☐
Other illness, health problems or medical conditions not listed.	☐	☐

Explanation of items marked "Yes":
_____
_____
_____

I certify that the medical information I have given is complete and accurate. _____ Initials

For Internal Use Only Below This Line
_____
_____
_____

Skin Analysis Form

Name:_____ DOB: _____

Date of last skin treatment and type:_____

Reported skin type: Normal Dry Combination Oily Acneic Sensitive Rosacea Other: _____

Allergic to: Sulfa   Milk Aloe Aspirin Grapes   Apples   Citrus   Shellfish   Other: _____

Reaction: _____

Current Regimen: _____

Specific Complaints: _____

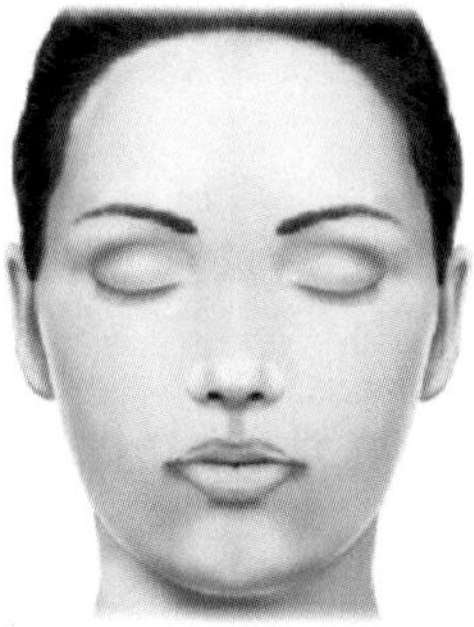

_____ Fitzpatrick Skin Type

_____ Glogau

W - Wrinkles	PP - Papules/ Pustules	C - Comedones	M - Milia
HP - Hyperpigmentation	T - Telangiectasias	ER - Erythema	SC - Scarring
HYP - Hypopigmentation	S - Scaling	LP - Large Pores	O - Oiliness

Observations: _____

Assessment: _____

Treatment Plan

Topical Products: _____

In-Office Treatments: _____

☐ Risks, benefits, alternatives and complications of Skin Care Treatments discussed with patient and all questions were answered

☐ Skin Care Consent signed and placed in chart

☐ Photographs taken

Signature: _____ Date: _____

Consent for Skin Care Treatments

This consent form provides the necessary information to assist patients in making an informed decision regarding receiving Skin Care Treatments that include, but are not limited to, microdermabrasion, chemical peels, and the use of topical skin care products.

Microdermabrasion is a mechanical method of removing the outermost layers of the skin through the use of abrasive elements such as a diamond-tipped pad. Chemical peels remove the top layers of the skin through the use of acids, such as glycolic, lactic, salicylic, and trichloroacetic acid.

Alternative treatments to microdermabrasion and chemical peels include laser skin resurfacing, dermabrasion, plastic surgery, or no treatment at all.

Possible risks, side effects, and complications with Skin Care Treatments include, but are not limited to:

- Prolonged erythema (redness) or edema (swelling)
- Allergic reactions
- Blistering
- Visible flaking/peeling
- Hyperpigmentation or hypopigmentation
- Abrasion (superficial cut) or temporary lines and streaking may occur with micro-dermabrasion
- Acne outbreak or the activation of recurrent viral infections such as herpes simplex may occur
- Infection or scarring

The risks of complications are higher for patients with darker skin types. I have disclosed any condition that may have bearing on this procedure such as: pregnancy, recent facial surgery, allergies, tendency to cold sores/fever blisters, or use of topical and/or oral prescription medications.

I understand that it is not possible to predict any of the above side effects or complications, and results are not guaranteed. I have fully read this consent form and understand the information provided to me regarding the proposed procedures, and I have had all questions and concerns answered to my satisfaction.

Patient Name _____   _____

Patient Signature _____   Date _____

Witness _____   Date _____

Before and After Instructions for Skin Care Treatments

Prior to Treatment

- Avoid tanning and direct sun exposure for 2 weeks prior to each treatment.
- Apply a sunscreen with SPF 30 or greater everyday for the duration of treatments.
- Apply topical products as instructed prior to treatment to prepare the skin.
- Discontinue use of any products containing high strength alpha hydroxy acids (such as glycolic and lactic acids) and prescription retinoids (such as Retin-A and Renova) 1–2 weeks prior to treatment.
- Consult with your personal physician before starting treatment if any skin lesions in the treatment areas have changed, itched, or bled.
- Treatment areas must be free of any open sores, lesions, or skin infections.
- If receiving chemical peels, only one chemical peel may be performed in a 2-week period.

After Treatment

- Treated areas may feel sensitive, tight, or dry and may appear pink, red, and slightly swollen for 3–5 days.
- Discomfort is rare, and may be alleviated with an over-the-counter pain reliever such as acetaminophen (Tylenol) or with the use of a cool compress 15 minutes every hour a few times per day.
- After the chemical peel procedure, skin may peel to varying degrees (mild, hardly visible, or heavy continuous peeling) depending on the treatment received and the condition of the skin prior to treatment. Peeling may last up to 2 weeks.
- Avoid becoming overheated, perspiring excessively, using hot tubs, steam rooms, saunas, or excessively hot showers in the first few days after treatment, as this can cause blistering and increase the risk of complications.
- Apply any postprocedure topical products as instructed. Regular home skin care products (including alpha hydroxy and retinoic acids) may be resumed 1–2 weeks after treatment or as instructed. Moisturizer may be applied twice a day or more frequently as needed for hydration and to decrease the appearance of flaking.
- During the healing process, avoid picking, scrubbing, exfoliating, or abrading sensitive or peeling skin as this may result in irritation and increase the risk of pigmentation changes and scarring.
- Mineral makeup may be applied after the treatment if desired. It is preferable to apply makeup the day following treatment.
- Avoid direct sun exposure and tanning bed use for 2–4 weeks after treatment and use a broad-spectrum sunscreen with SPF 30 or greater containing zinc or titanium daily.
- Avoid hot tubs, swimming, and other water activities for 2 weeks.
- Avoid electrolysis, facial waxing, or the use of depilatories for 2 weeks after treatment.

Skin Care Procedure Notes

Name:_____   DOB:_____   Fitz:_____

       Last,   First

Date:	Tx Area:	MDA:			
Skin Complaints:		Grit/Vacuum(psi)			
		Serum/Infusion (mL/min)			
Pre Tx Observations:		# Passes			
Treatment:		Chemical Peels:	Peel 1:	Peel 2:	Peel 3:
Skin Prep:		Acid, %			
		# Layers			
		Time (min)			
Enzyme (min):		Notes:			
Extractions: Yes / No					
Treatment Serum:		Response from this tx: □ erythema: mild – mod – severe Areas ↑ erythema: _____			
Mask:		□ Petechiae: _____ □ Striping*: _____ □ Hives*: _____ □ Itchiness*: _____ □ Other:			
Serum:		Post Tx: □ Cold compress □ HC 1% / 2.5% / TAC 0.5% □ Other: _____			
Moisturizer/SPF:		□ See Home Skin Care Sheet □ Refer to Narrative Progress Notes* □ MD notified*			
		□ See Med and Allergy List □ Reviewed written post tx instructions **Signed by:**			
Date:	**Tx Area:**	**MDA:**			
Skin Complaints:		Grit/Vacuum(psi)			
		Serum/Infusion (mL/min)			
Pre Tx Observations:		# Passes			
Treatment:		Chemical Peels:	Peel 1:	Peel 2:	Peel 3:
Skin Prep:		Acid, %			
		# Layers			
		Time (min)			
Enzyme (min):		Notes:			
Extractions: Yes / No					
Treatment Serum:		Response from this tx: □ erythema: mild – mod – severe Areas ↑ erythema: _____			
Mask:		□ Petechiae: _____ □ Striping*: _____ □ Hives*: _____ □ Itchiness*: _____ □ Other:			
Serum:		Post Tx: □ Cold compress □ HC 1% / 2.5% / TAC 0.5% □ Other: _____			
Moisturizer/SPF:		□ See Home Skin Care Sheet □ Refer to Narrative Progress Notes* □ MD notified*			
		□ See Med and Allergy List □ Reviewed written post tx instructions **Signed by:**			
Date:	**Tx Area:**	**MDA:**			
Skin Complaints:		Grit/Vacuum(psi)			
		Serum/Infusion (mL/min)			
Pre Tx Observations:		# Passes			
Treatment:		Chemical Peels:	Peel 1:	Peel 2:	Peel 3:
Skin Prep:		Acid, %			
		# Layers			
		Time (min)			
Enzyme (min):		Notes:			
Extractions: Yes / No					
Treatment Serum:		Response from this tx: □ erythema: mild – mod – severe Areas ↑ erythema: _____			
Mask:		□ Petechiae: _____ □ Striping*: _____ □ Hives*: _____ □ Itchiness*: _____ □ Other:			
Serum:		Post Tx: □ Cold compress □ HC 1% / 2.5% / TAC 0.5% □ Other: _____			
Moisturizer/SPF:		□ See Home Skin Care Sheet □ Refer to Narrative Progress Notes* □ MD notified*			
		□ See Med and Allergy List □ Reviewed written post tx instructions **Signed by:**			

Microdermabrasion Supply Sources

Altair Instruments
Phone: 1-866-325-8247
www.diamondtome.com

Aesthetic Technologies
Phone: 1-408-464-8893
www.mmizone.com

Bella Products
Phone: 1-877-550-5655
www.bellaproducts.com

Bio-Therapeutic
Phone: 1-800-976-2544
www.bio-therapeutic.com

DermaSweep
Phone: 1-916-632-9134
www.dermasweep.com

DermaMed International
Phone: 1-888-789-6342
www.megapeel.com

DermaTone USA
Phone: 1-800-289-1574
www.dermatoneusa.com

DermaVista
Phone: 1-800-333-5773
www.dermavista.com

Dynatronics
Phone: 1-800-874-6251
www.dynatronics.com

Edge Systems
Phone: 1-800-603-4996
www.edgesystem.net

Envy Medical
Phone: 1-888-848-3633
www.silkpeel.com

ExcellaDerm
Phone: 1-877-969-7546
www.excelladerm.com

Lumenis
Phone: 1-408-764-3000
www.lumenis.com

Marketech International (Dermagrain)
Phone: 1-877-452-4910
www.dermagrain.com

Mattioli Engineering (Ultrapeel)
Phone: 1-703-312-6000
www.mattioliengineering.com

Med-Aesthetic Solutions
Phone: 1-877-733-7627
www.medaestheticsolutions.com

RAJA Medical
Phone: 1-877-880-4184
www.rajamedical.com

Silhouet-Tone USA
Phone: 1-800-463-2710
www.silhouet-tone.com

Sybaritic
Phone: 1-800-445-8418
www.sybaritic.com

Syneron
Phone: 1-866-259-6661
www.syneron.com

Chemical Peel and Topical Product Supply Sources

TABLE 1

Chemical Peels

Company Name	AHA	BHA	TCA	Jessner's	Blended	Retinoid
Allergan	X					
California Skincare Supply (D)	X	X		X	X	X
Circadia	X	X		X	X	X
DermaQuest	X	X	X	X	X	X
Global Skin Solutions	X	X		X	X	
GlyMed Plus	X	X	X	X	X	X
Glytone	X	X	X			
Jan Marini	X					
Medicalia	X				X	
Mesoestetic USA	X	X			X	
Neostrata Company	X					
Obagi			X		X	
PCA SKIN	X	X	X	X	X	X
Rhonda Allison	X	X	(X)	X	X	X
SkinCeuticals	X	X		X	X	
SkinMedica					X	X
Topix Pharmaceuticals (D)	X			X		
University Specialty Pharmacy						X

AHA = Alpha hydroxy acid; BHA = Beta hydroxy acid; TCA = Trichloroacetic acid; D = Distributor; (X) = Currently unavailable.

TABLE 2

Topical Products

Company Name	Sunscreen[a]	Indications				
		Photoaging	Erythema[b]	Acne	Hyperpigmentation	Postprocedure
Allergan	X	X			X	X
Cellex-C	X	X	X	X	X	
Circadia	X	X	X	X	X	X
CosmMedix	X	X	X	X	X	X
DermaQuest	X	X	X	X	X	X
EltaMD Skincare	X					
Fallene	X					
Galderma	X	X		X	X	
Galderma Labs.	X		X			
Global Skin Soln.	X	X		X	X	X
GlyMed Plus	X	X	X	X	X	X
Glytone	X	X				
iS CLINICAL	X	X	X	X	X	
Jan Marini	X	X		X	X	
Kinerase		X	X	X		
Medicalia	X	X	X	X	X	
Neostrata	X	X		X	X	
Neutrogena	X	X	X	X	X	
NIA 24	X	X	X		X	X
Obagi	X	X	X	X	X	
PCA SKIN	X	X	X	X	X	X
ResultsRx	X	X	X	X	X	X
Rhonda Allison	X	X	X	X	X	X
SkinCeuticals	X	X	X	X	X	X
SkinMedica	X	X	X	X		X
Valeant Pharm.	X		X			

[a]Sunscreen refers to broad-spectrum sunscreen products of SPF 30 or greater.
[b]Erythema refers to facial erythema associated with rosacea and sensitive skin.

Allergan
Phone: 1-800-433-8871
www.allergan.com

Biopelle
Phone: 1-866-424-6735
www.biopelle.com

California Skincare Supply, Inc.
Phone: 1-800-500-1886
www.californiaskincaresupply.com

Cellex-C
Phone: 1-888-409-9979
www.cellex-c.com

Circadia
Phone: 1-800-630-4710
www.circadia.com

DermaQuest
Phone: 1-800-213-8100
www.dermaquestinc.com

EltaMD Skincare
Phone: 1-800-633-8872
www.eltamd.com

Fallene
Phone: 1-800-332-5536
www.fallene.com

Galderma Laboratories
Phone: 1-866-735-4137
www.galderma.com

Global Skin Solutions
Phone: 1-623-486-1234
www.pamelaspringer.com

GlyMed Plus
1-801-798-0390
www.glymedplus.com

Glytone
Phone: 1-800-459-8663
www.glytone-usa.com

iS CLINICAL
Phone: 888-807-4447
www.isclinical.com

Jan Marini Skin
Phone: 1-800-347-2223
www.janmarini.com

Kinerase
Phone: 1-800-321-4576
www.kinerase.com

Merz Pharmaceuticals
Phone: 1-877-MERZUSA
www.merzusa.com

Mesoestetic USA
Phone: 818-783-6881
www.mesoesteticusa.com

Neostrata Company
Phone: 1-800-225-9411
www.neostrata.com

NIA 24
Phone: 1-866-NIADYNE
www.nia24.com

Obagi
Phone: 562-628-1007
www.obagi.com

PCA SKIN
Phone: 877-722-7546
www.pcaskin.com

Rhonda Allison
Phone: 866-313-7546
www.rhondaallison.com

Sederma
www.sederma.fr

SkinCeuticals
Phone: 1-800-811-1660
www.skinceuticals.com

SkinMedica
Phone: 1-866-867-0110
www.skinmedica.com

Topix Pharmaceuticals
Phone: 1-800-445-2595
www.topixpharm.com

University Specialty Pharmacy
Phone: 323-2024488
www.universitysp.com

Valeant Pharmaceuticals
Phone: 1-800-548-5100
www.valeant.com

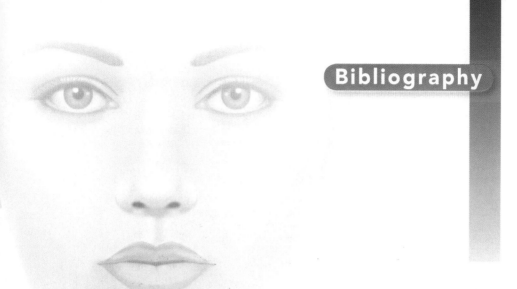

Aesthetic Procedure Statistics and Overview

Cosmetic Surgery National Data Bank Statistics 2011. American Society for Aesthetic Plastic Surgery. http://www.surgery.org/media/statistics. Accessed on September 19, 2012.
Small R. Aesthetic Procedures in Office Practice. Am Fam Physician. 2009;80(11):1231–1237.

Skin Anatomy

Downie JB. Esthetic considerations for ethnic skin. Semin Cutan Med Surg. 2006;25:158–162.
Netter FH. Atlas of Human Anatomy. 4th ed. Philadelphia, PA. Saunders. 2006;24(25):35–50.
Pouillot A, Dayan N, Polla A, et al. The Stratum Corneum: a double paradox. J Cosmet Dermatol. 2008;7:139–142.

Consultation

Fitzpatrick TB. The validity and practicality of sun-reactive skin types I through VI. Arch Dermatol. 1988;124(6):869–871.
Glogau RG. Aesthetic and anatomic analysis of the aging skin. Semin Cutan Med Surg. 1996;15(3):134–138.
Small R. Aesthetic Principles and Consultation. In: Usatine R, Pfenninger J, Stulberg D, and Small R, eds. Dermatologic and Cosmetic Procedures in Office Practice. Philadelphia, PA. Elsevier. 2011:230–239.
Small R. Aesthetic Procedures Introduction. In: Mayeaux E, ed. The Essential Guide to Primary Care Procedures. Philadelphia, PA. Lippincott Williams & Wilkins. 2009:195–199.

Photoaging

Choudhary S, Tang JC, Leiva A, et al. Photodamage, Part 1: Pathophysiology, Clinical Manifestations, and Photoprotection. Cosmet Dermatol. 2010;23:460–466.
Choudhary S, Tang J, Leiva A, et al. Photodamage, Part 2: Management of photoaging. Cosmet Dermatol. 2010;23(11):496–509.
Fisher GJ, Kang S, Varani J, et al. Mechanisms of photoaging and chronological skin aging. Arch Dermatol. 2002;138:1462–1470.
Lockman AR, Lockman DW. Skin changes in the maturing woman. Clinics in Family Practice. 2002;4(1):113–134.
Lowe NJ, Meyers DP, Wieder JM. Low doses of repetitive ultraviolet A induce morphologic changes in human skin. J Invest Dermatol. 1995;105:739–743.
Rabe JH, Mamelak AJ, McElgunn PJS, et al. Photoaging: mechanisms and repair. J Am Acad Dermatol. 2006;55:1–19.
Samuel M, Brooke RC, Hollis S, et al. Review Interventions for photodamaged skin. Cochrane Database Syst Rev. 2005;(1):CD001782.

Chemical Peels

Overview

Clark CP. Office-based skin care and superficial peels: The scientific rationale. Plast Reconstr Surg. 1999;104(3):854–864.
Clark E, Scerri L. Superficial and medium-depth chemical peels. Clin Dermatol. 2008;26(2):209–218.
Drake LA, Dinehart SM, Goltz RW, et al. Guidelines of care for chemical peeling. Guidelines/Outcomes Committee: American Academy of Dermatology. J Am Acad Dermatol. 1995;33:479–503.
Dugas B. Choosing the right peel for your patient. Plast Surg Nurs. 2007;27:80–84.

Fischer TC, Perosino E, Poli F, et al. Chemical peels in aesthetic dermatology: an update 2009. J Eur Acad Dermatol Venereol. 2010;24(3):281–292.

Khunger N. Standard guidelines for chemical peels. Indian J Dermatol Venereol Leprol. 2008;74:S5–S12.

Landau M. Chemical peels. Clin Dermatol. 2008;26:200–208.

Linder J. Superficial Chemical Peeling: Minimal Effort, Maximum Results. Skin & Aging. 2011;19:32–36.

Mangat D, Tansavatdi K, Garlich P. Current chemical peels and other resurfacing techniques. Facial Plast Surg. 2011;27:35–49.

Matarasso SL, Glogau RG. Chemical face peels. Dermatol Clin. 1991;9(1):131–150.

Matarasso SL, Salman SM, Glogau RG, et al. The role of chemical peeling in the treatment of photodamaged skin. J Dermatol Surg Oncol. 1990;16:945–954.

Monheit GD. Chemical Peels. Skin Therapy Lett. 2004;9:6–11.

Roberts WE. Chemical peeling in ethnic/darker skin. Dermatol Ther. 2004;17:196–205.

Small R, O'Hanlon K. Chemical Peels. In: Usatine R, Pfenninger J, Stulberg D, and Small R, eds. Dermatologic and Cosmetic Procedures in Office Practice. Philadelphia, PA. Elsevier. 2011:259–273.

Zakapoulu N, Kontochistopoulous G. Superficial chemical peels. J Cosmet Dermatol. 2006;5(3):246–253.

Treatment

Alpha Hydroxy Acid Peels

Bergfeld WF, Tung RC, Vidimos AT. Improving the appearance of photoaged skin with glycolic acid. J Am Acad Dermatol. 1997;36:1011–1013.

Briden M. Alpha-hydroxyacid chemical peeling agents: Case studies and rationale for safe and effective use. Cutis. 2004;73:18–24.

Murad H, Shamban AT, Premo PS. The use of glycolic acid as a peeling agent. Dermatol Clin. 1995;13: 285–307.

Sehgal V, Luthra A, Aggerwal A. Evaluation of graded strength glycolic acid facial peel: an Indian experience. J Dermatol. 2003;30(758):761.

Slavin JW. Considerations in alpha hydroxy acid peels. Clin Plast Surg. 1998;25:45–52.

Salicylic Acid Peels

Bari AU, Iqbal Z, Rahman SB. Tolerance and safety of superficial chemical peeling with salicylic acid in various facial dermatoses. Indian J Dermatol Venereol Leprol. 2005;71:87–90.

Grimes PE. The safety and efficacy of salicylic acid chemical peels in darker racial-ethnic groups. Derm Surg. 1999;25:18–22.

Kligman D, Kligman AM. Salicylic acid peels for the treatment of photoaging. Dermatol Surg. 1998;24: 325–328.

Krunic A, Cetner A, Grimes P. Salicylic acid peels - our experience with dyschromia, photoaging and acne-related conditions. Kosmetische Medizin. 2007;28:173–175.

Moy LS, Murad H, Moy RL. Glycolic acid peels for the treatment of wrinkles and photoaging. J Dermatol Surg Oncol. 1993;19:243–246.

Vedamurthy M. Salicylic acid peels. Indian J Dermatol Venereol Leprol. 2004;70:136–138.

Trichloroacetic Acid Peels

Nguyen TH, Rooney JA. Trichloroacetic acid peels. Dermatol Ther. 2000;13:173–182.

Slavin JW. Trichloroacetic acid peels. Aesthetic Surg J. 2004;24:469–470.

Jessner's Peels

Fulton JE. Jessner's Peel. In: Rubin MG, Dover JS, and Alam M, eds. Procedures in Cosmetic Dermatology: Chemical Peels. Philadelphia, PA. Elsevier Saunders. 2006:57–72.

Lawrence N, Cox SE, Brody HJ. Treatment of melasma with Jessner's solution versus glycolic acid: a comparison of clinical efficacy and evaluation of the predictive ability of Wood's light examination. Am Acad Dermatol. 1977;36:589–593.

Retinoid Peels

Cuce L, Bertino M, Scattone L, et al. Tretinoin peeling. Derm Surg. 2001;27:12–14.

Khunger N, Sarkar R, Jain RK. Tretinoin peels versus glycolic acid peels in the treatment of Melasma in dark-skinned patients. Derm Surg. 2004;30(5):756–760.

Blended Peels

Coleman WP, Futrell JM. The glycolic acid trichloroacetic acid peel. J Dermatol Surg Oncol. 1994;20:76–80.

Ellis DAF, Tan AKW, Ellis CS. Superficial micropeels: Glycolic acid and alpha-hydroxy acid with kojic acid. Facial Plast Surg. 1995;11:15–21.

Microdermabrasion

Bhalla M, Thami GP. Microdermabrasion: reappraisal and brief review of literature. Derm Surg. 2006;32(6): 809–814.

Coimbra M, Rohrich RJ, Chao J, et al. A prospective controlled assessment of microdermabrasion for damaged skin and fine rhytides. Plast Reconstr Surg. 2004;113(5):1438–1443.

Comite SL, Krishtal A, Tan MH. Using microdermabrasion to treat sun-induced facial lentigines and photoaging. Cosmetic Dermatol. 2003;16:40–42.

Desai TD, Moy R. Evaluation of the SilkPeel system in treating erythematotelangectatic and papulopustular rosacea. Cosm Derm. 2006;19(1):51–57.

Freedman BM, Rueda-Pedraza E, Waddell S. The epidermal and dermal changes associated with microdermabrasion. Derm Surg. 2001;27(12):1031–1034.

Freeman MS. Microdermabrasion. Facial Plast Surg Clin North Am. 2001;9(2):257–266.

Grimes P. Microdermabrasion. Derm Surg. 2005;31(9):1160–1165.

Hernandez-Perez E, Ibiett EV. Gross and microscopic findings in patients undergoing microdermabrasion for facial rejuvenation. Derm Surg. 2001;27(7):637–640.

Karimipour DJ, Kang S, Johnson T, et al. Microdermabrasion with and without aluminum oxide crystal abrasion: A comparative molecular analysis of dermal remodeling. J Am Acad Derm. 2006;54(3):405–410.

Koch RJ, Hanasono M. Microdermabrasion. Facial Plast Surg Clin of N Am. 2001;9(3):377–381.

Lew BK, Cho Y, Lee M. Effect of serial microdermabrasion on the ceramide level in the stratum corneum. Dermatol Surg. 2006;32:376–379.

Rajan P, Grimes PE. Skin barrier changes induced by aluminum oxide and sodium chloride microdermabrasion. Derm Surg. 2002;28(5):390–393.

Rubin MG, Greenbaum SS. Histologic effects of almumin oxide microdermabrasion on facial skin. J Aesth Derm Cosmetic Surg. 2000;I:237.

Sadick N. A review of microdermabrasion. Cosm Derm. 2005;18:351–354.

Small R. Microdermabrasion. In: Mayeaux E, ed. The Essential Guide to Primary Care Procedures. Philadelphia, PA. Lippincott Williams & Wilson. 2009:265–277.

Small R, Quema R. Microdermabrasion. In: Usatine R, Pfenninger J, Stulberg D, and Small R, eds. Dermatologic and Cosmetic Procedures in Office Practice. Philadelphia, PA. Elsevier. 2011:274–283.

Tsai RY, Wang CN, Chan HL. Aluminum oxide crystal microdermabrasion. A new technique for treating facial scarring. Derm Surg. 1995;21:539–542.

Topical Products

Overview

Chiu A, Kimball AB. Topical vitamins, minerals and botanical ingredients as modulators of environmental and chronological skin damage. Brit J Dermatol. 2003;149:681–691.

Draelos Z. The latest cosmeceutical approaches for anti-aging. J Cosmet Dermatol. 2007;6:2–6.

Linder J. Cosmeceutical Treatment of the Aging Face. In: Prendergast PM, Shiffman MA, eds. Aesthetic Medicine Art and Techniques. Spinger Berlin Heidelberg. 2011:69–84.

Small R, Green B. Skin Care Products. In: Usatine R, Pfenninger J, Stuhlberg D, and Small R, eds. Dermatologic and Cosmetic Procedures in Office Practice. Philadelphia, PA. Elsevier. 2011:286–297.

Treatment

Growth Factors

Atkin DH, Trookman NS, Rizer RL, et al. Combination of physiologically balanced growth factors with antioxidants for reversal of facial photodamage. J Cosmet Laser Ther. 2010;12(1):14–20.

Fitzpatrick RE, Rostan EF. Reversal of photodamage with topical growth factors: a pilot study. J Cosmet Laser Ther. 2003;5(1):25–34.

Fitzpatrick RE. Endogenous growth factors as cosmeceuticals. Derm Surg. 2005;31:827–831.

Mehta RC, Smith SR, Grove GL, et al. Reduction in facial photodamage by a topical growth factor product. J Drugs Dermatol. 2008;7(9):864–871.

Rattan SI. N6-furfuryladenine (Kinetin) as a potential anti-aging molecule. J Anti-Aging Medicine. 2002;5(1):113–116.

Rattan SI, Sodagam L. Gerontomodulatory and youth-preserving effects of zeatin on human skin fibroblasts undergoing aging *in vitro*. Rejuvenation Res. 2005;8(1):46–57.

Retinoids

Creidi P, Humbert P. Clinical use of topical retinaldehyde on photoaged skin. Dermatology. 1999;199 (suppl 1):49–52.

Darlenski R, Surber C, Fluhr JW. Topical Retinoids in the Management of Photodamaged Skin: From Theory to Evidence-based Practical Approach. Brit J Derm. 2010;163(6):1157–1165.

Draelos ZD. Retinoids in cosmetics. Cosmet Dermatol. 2005;18:3–5.

Farris PK, Rendon MI. The mechanism of action of topical retinoids for the treatment of nonmalignant photodamage, part 1. Cosmet Dermatol. 2010;23(1):19–24.

Hamerlynck JV, Middeldorp S, Scholten RJ. Improvement of photodamaged skin with retinoid creams and not with other local treatments Review From the Cochrane Library. Ned Tijdschr Geneeskd. 2006;150(3):140–142.

Kafi R, Kwak HS, Schumacher WE, et al. Improvement of naturally aged skin with vitamin A (retinol). Arch Dermatol. 2007;143(5):606–612.

Kang S, Duell EA, Fisher GJ, Datta SC, et al. Application of retinol to human skin in vivo induces epidermal hyperplasia and cellular retinoid binding proteins characteristic of retinoic acid but without measurable retinoic acid levels or irritation. J Invest Dermatol. 1995;105:549–556.

Kligman A, Grove GL, Hirose E, et al. Topical tretinoin for photoaged skin. J Am Acad Dermatol. 1986;15:836–859.

Lew BL, Cho Y, Lee MH. Effect of serial microdermabrasion on the ceramide level in the stratum corneum. Derm Surg. 2006;32:376–379.

Lloyd JR. The use of microdermabrasion for acne: a pilot study. Dermatol Surg. 2001;27:329–331.

Machtinger LA, Kaidbey K, Lim J, et al. Histologic effects of tazarotene 0.1% cream vs. vehicle on photodamaged skin: a 6 month multicenter, double-blind, randomized, vehicle-controlled study in patients with photodamaged facial skin. Brit J Derm. 2004;151:1245–1252.

Rolewski SL. Clinical review: Topical retinoids. Dermatol Nurs. 2003;15:447–465.

Sachsenberg-Studer EM. Tolerance of topical retinaldehyde in humans. Dermatology. 1999;199(suppl 1):61–63.

Singh M, Griffiths CE. The use of retinoids in the treatment of photoaging. Dermatol Ther. 2006;19(5):297–305.

Stratigos AJ, Katsambas AD. The role of topical retinoids in the treatment of photoaging. Drugs. 2005;65:1061–1072.

Ting W. Tretinoin for the treatment of photodamaged skin. Cutis. 2010;86(1):47–52.

Tucker-Samaras S, Zedayko T, Cole C, et al. A Stabilized 0.1% Retinol Facial Moisturizer Improves the Appearance of Photodamaged Skin in an Eight-Week, Double-Blind, Vehicle-Controlled Study Source. J Drugs Dermatol. 2009;8(10):932–936.

Weinstein GD, Nigra TP, Pochi PE, et al. Topical tretinoin for treatment of photodamaged skin: a multicenter study. Arch Dermatol. 1991;127:659–665.

Moisturizers

Del Rosso JQ. Moisturizers: function, formulation and clinical applications. In: Draelos Z, Dover JS, and Alam M, eds. Procedures in Cosmetic Dermatology: Cosmeceuticals. Philadelphia, PA. Saunders Elsevier. 2009:97–101.

Kraft BN, Lynde CW. Moisturizers: What they are and a practical approach to product selection. Skin Therapy Lett. 2005;10:1–8.

Rawlings AV, Harding CR. Moisturization and skin barrier function. Dermatol Ther. 2004;17:43–48.

Hydroxy Acids

Berardesca E, Distante F, Vignoli GP, et al. Alpha hydroxyacids modulate stratum corneum barrier function. Brit J Dermatol. 1997;137:934–938.

Bernstein EF, Lee J, Brown DB, et al. Glycolic acid treatment increases type I collagen mRNA and hyaluronic acid content of human skin. Derm Surg. 2001;27(5):429–433.

Bernstein EF, Underhill CB, Lakkakorpi J, et al. Citric acid increases viable epidermal thickness and glycosaminoglycan content of sun-damaged skin. Derm Surg. 1997;23(8):689–694.

Ditre CM, Griffin TD, Murphy GF, et al. Effects of alpha hydroxyacids on photoaged skin: a pilot clinical, histological and ultrastructural study. J Am Acad Dermatol. 1996;34:187–195.

Green BA, Edison BL, Singler ML. Antiaging effects of topical lactobionic acid: results of a controlled usage study. Cosmet Dermatol. 2008;21(2):76–82.

Green BA, Yu RJ, Van Scott EJ. Clinical and cosmeceutical uses of hydroxyacids. Clinics in Dermatology. 2009;27(5):495–501.

Rawlings AV, Davies A, Carlomusto M. Effect of lactic acid isomers on keratinocyte ceramide synthesis, stratum corneum lipid levels and stratum corneum barrier function. Arch Dermatol. 1996;288:383–390.

Van Scott EJ, Yu RJ. Hyperkeratinization, corneocyte cohesion and alpha hydroxy acids. J Am Acad Dermatol. 1984;11:867–879.

Niacinamide

Bissett DL, Miyamoto K, Sun P, et al. Topical niacinamide reduces yellowing, wrinkling, red blotchiness, and hyperpigmented spots in aging facial skin. Int J Cosmet Sci. 2004;26:231–238.

Bissett DL, Robinson LR, Raleigh P, et al. Reduction in the appearance of facial hyperpigmentation by topical N-undecyl-10-enoyl-L-phenylalanine and its combination with niacinamide. J Cosmet Dermatol. 2009;8:260–266.

Gehring W. Nicotinic acid/niacinamide and the skin. J Cosmet Dermatol. 2004;3:88–93.

Peptides

Blanes-Mira C, Clemente J, Jodas G, et al. A synthetic hexapeptide (Argireline) with antiwrinkle activity. Int J Cos Sci. 2002;24:303–310.

Fields K, Falla TJ, Rodan K, et al. Bioactive peptides: signaling the future. J Cosmet Dermatol. 2009;8:8–13.

Katayama K, rmendariz-Borunda J, Raghow R, et al. A pentapeptide from type I procollagen promotes extracellular matrix production. J Biol Chem. 1993;268:9941–9944.

Lupo MP, Cole AL. Cosmeceutical peptides. Dermatol Ther. 2007;20:343–349.

Metalloprotease Inhibitors

Tanaka K, Asamitsu K, Uranishi H, et al. Protecting skin photoaging by NF-kappaB inhibitor. Curr Drug Metab. 2010:11(5):431–435.
Thibodeau A. Metalloproteinase inhibitors. Cosmet Toil. 2000;115(11):75–76.

Amino Sugars

Bissett DL. Glucosamine: An ingredient with skin and other benefits. J Cosmet Dermatol. 2006;5:309–315.
Mammone T, Gan D, Fthenakis C. The effect of N-acetyl-glucosamine on stratum corneum desquamation and water content in human skin. J Cosmet Sci. 2009;60:423–428.

Protect

Antioxidants

Baxter R. Anti-aging properties of resveratrol: review and report of a potent new antioxidant skin care formulation. J Cosmet Dermatol. 2008;7:2–7.
Farris PK. Topical vitamin C: a useful agent for treating photoaging and other dermatologic conditions. Dermatol Surg. 2005;31:814–817.
Fitzpatrick RE, Rostan EF. Double-blind, half-face study comparing topical vitamin C and vehicle for rejuvenation of photodamage. Derm Surg. 2002;28(3):231–236.
Haywood R, Wardman P, Saunders R, et al. Sunscreens inadequately protect against ultraviolet-A-induced free radicals in skin: implications for skin aging and melanoma? J Invest Dermatol. 2003;121:862–868.
Katiyar SK. Silymarin and skin cancer prevention: Anti-inflammatory, antioxidant and immunomodulatory effects. Int J Oncol. 2005;26:1213–1222.
Lin FH, Lin JY, Gupta RD, et al. Ferulic acid stabilizes a solution of vitamins C and E and doubles its photoprotection of skin. J Invest Dermatol. 2005;125:826–832.
Linder J. Antioxidants: Crucial Additions to Dermal Photoprotection. Cosmetic Dermatology. 2010;23:40–44.
Lupo MP, Draelos ZD, Farris P, et al. CoffeeBerry: A new, natural antioxidant in professional anti-aging skin care. Cosmet Dermatol. 2007;20:1–9.
Nusgens BV, Humbert P, Rougier A, et al. Topically applied vitamin C enhances the mRNA level of collagens I and III, their processing enzymes and tissue inhibitor of matrix metalloproteinase 1 in the human dermis. J Invest Dermatol. 2001;116:853–859.
Pinnell SR. Regulation of collagen biosynthesis by ascorbic acid: a review. Yale J Biol Med. 1985;58: 553–559.
Placzek M, Gaube S, Kerkmann U, et al. Ultraviolet B-induced DNA damage in human epidermis is modified by the antioxidants ascorbic acid and D-α-tocopherol. J Invest Dermatol. 2005;124:304–307.
Tournas JA, Lin FH, Burch J, et al. Ubiquinone, idebenone, and kinetin provide ineffective photoprotection to skin when compared to a topical antioxidant combination of vitamins C and E with ferulic acid. J Invest Dermatol. 2006;126:1185–1187.
Zhai H, Cordoba-Diaz M, Wa C, et al. Determination of the antioxidant capacity of an antioxidant complex and idebenone: an *in vitro* rapid and sensitive method. J Cosmet Dermatol. 2008;7:96–100.

Sunscreens

Hawk JL. Cutaneous photoprotection. Arch Dermatol. 2003;139:527–530.
Fourtanier A, Moyal D, Seite S. UVA filters in sun-protection products: regulatory and biological aspects. Photochem Photobiol Sci. 2012;11(1):81–89.
Sambandan DR, Ratner D. Sunscreens: An overview and update. J Am Acad Dermatol. 2011;64:748–758.
Sayre RM, Kollias N, Roberts RL, et al. Physical sunscreens. J Soc Cosmet Chem. 1990;41:103–109.

Facial Erythema

Overview

Blount BW, Pelletier AL. Rosacea: A common, yet commonly overlooked, condition. Am Fam Physician. 2002;66:435–441.
Crawford GH, Pelle MT, James WD. Rosacea: I. Etiology, pathogenesis, and subtype classification. J Am Acad Dermatol. 2004;51(3):327–341.

Treatment

Baumann LS. Cosmeceutical critique: allantoin. Skin & Allergy News. 2003;34:10.
Baumann LS. Cosmeceutical critique: aloe vera. Skin & Allergy News. 2003;34:32.
Baumann LS. Cosmeceutical critique: chamomile. Skin & Allergy News. 2003;39:43.
Emer J, Waldorf H, Berson D. Botanicals and anti-inflammatories: natural ingredients for rosacea. Semin Cutan Med Surg. 2011;30(3):148–155.

Draelos Z. Optimizing redness reduction, Part 1: Roscacea and skin care. Cosmet Dermatol. 2008;21(7): 383–386.

Draelos Z. Optimizing redness reduction, Part 2: Rosacea and cosmeceuticals. Cosmet Dermatol. 2008;21(8): 433–436.

Hsu S. Green tea and the skin. J Am Acad Derm. 2005;52:1049–1059.

Thornfeldt C. Cosmeceuticals containing herbs: fact, fiction, and future. Dermatol Surg. 2005;31(7):873–880.

Tollesson A, Frithz A. Borage oil. an effective new treatment for infantile seborrhoeic dermatitis. Br J Dermatol. 1993;129:95.

Van Zuuren EJ, Kramer SF, Carter BR, et al. Effective and evidence-based management strategies for rosacea: summary of a Cochrane systematic review. Br J Dermatol. 2011;165(4):760–781.

Acne

Overview

Goulden V, Clark SM, Cunliffe WJ. Post-adolescent acne: a review of clinical features. Br J Dermatol. 1997;136:66.

Jeremy AH, Holland DB, Roberts SG, et al. Inflammatory events are involved in acne lesion initiation. J Invest Dermatol. 2003;121:20.

Treatment

Del Rosso JQ. Topical retinoids in the management of acne: the best path to clear results. Cutis. 2004;74(4 suppl):2–3.

Kempiak SJ, Uebelhoer N. Superficial Chemical Peels and Microdermabrasion for Acne Vulgaris. Semin Cutan Med Surg. 2008;27:212–220.

Kessler E, Flanagan K, Chia C, et al. Comparison of alpha- and beta-hydroxy acid chemical peels in the treatment of mild to moderately severe facial acne vulgaris. Derm Surg. 2008;34(1):45–50.

Lee SH, Huh CH, Park KC, et al. Effects of repetitive superficial chemical peels on facial sebum secetion in acne patients. J Eur Acad Dermatol Venereol. 2006;20(8):964–968.

Lee HS, Kim IH. Salicylic acid peels for the treatment of acne vulgaris in Asian patients. Dermatol Surg. 2003;29:1196–1199; discussion 9.

Leyden JJ. A review of the use of combination therapies for the treatment of acne vulgaris. J Am Acad Dermatol. 2003;49:200–210.

Shalita AR, Chalker DK, Griffith RF, et al. Tazarotene gel is safe and effective in the treatment of acne vulgaris: a multicenter, double-blind, vehicle-controlled study. Cutis. 1999;63(6):349–354.

Strauss JS, Krowchuk DP, Leyden JJ, et al. Guidelines of care for acne vulgaris management. J Am Acad Dermatol. 2007;56:651–663.

Hyperpigmentation

Overview

Pandya A, Guevara I. Disorders of Hyperpigmentation. Dermatol Clin. 2000;18:91–98.

Pugliese PT. Physiology of the skin: pigmentation revisited. Skin Inc. 2009;21(3):68–76.

Yamaguchi Y, Brenner M, Hearing VJ. The regulation of skin pigmentation. J Biol Chem. 2007;282(38):27557–27561.

Treatment

Bissett DL, Robinson LR, Raleigh PS, et al. Reduction in the appearance of facial hyperpigmentation by topical N-acetyl glucosamine. J Cosmet Dermatol. 2007;6:20–26.

Draelos Z. Skin lightening challenges. Global Cosmetic Industry. 2009;2:40–44.

Kalla G, Garg A, Kachhawa D. Chemical peeling–glycolic acid versus trichloroacetic acid in melasma. Indian J Dermatol Venereol Leprol. 2001;67:82–84.

Khunger N, Sarkar R, Jain RK. Tretinoin peels versus glycolic acid peels in the treatment of melasma in dark-skinned patients. Dermatol Surg. 2004;30:756–760; discussion 60.

Linder J. Treatment Strategies for Challenging Melasma Cases. Skin & Aging. 2009;17:38–41.

Palm MD, Toombs EL. Hydroquinone and the FDA- the debate. J Drug Dermatol. 2007;6.2:122(1).

Rendon MI, Gaviria JI. Review of skin-lightening agents. Derm Surg. 2005;31:886–889.

Sharquie KE, Al-Tikreety MM, Al-Mashhadani SA. Lactic acid chemical peels as a new therapeutic modality in melasma in comparison to Jessner's solution chemical peels. Dermatol Surg. 2006;32:1429–1436.

Pre & Post Procedure Products

Nyriady J, Grossman R. Use of tretinoin in precosmetic and postcosmetic procedures: a review. Cosmet Dermatol. 2003;16:7–17.

Rendon MI, Cardona L, Benitez A. The safety and efficacy of trolamin/sodium algenate topical emulsion in postlaser resurfacing wounds. J Drugs Dermatol. 2008;7(5):S23–S28.

Tanzi EL, Perez M. The effect of a mucopolysaccharide-cartilage complex healing ointment on Er:YAG laser resurfaced facial skin. Dermatol Surg. 2002;28:305–308.

Combining Therapies

Briden ME, Jacobsen E, Johnson C. Combining superficial glycolic acid (alpha-hydroxy acid) peels with microdermabrasion to maximize treatment results and patient satisfaction. Cutis. 2007;79(1 suppl Combining):13–16.

Effron C, Briden ME, Green BA. Enhancing cosmetic outcomes by combining superficial glycolic acid (alpha-hydroxy acid) peels with nonablative lasers, intense pulsed light, and trichloroacetic acid peels. Cutis. 2007;79(1 suppl Combining):4–8.

Erbil H, Sezer E, Tastan B, el al. Efficacy and safety of serial glycolic acid peels and a topical regimen in the treatment of recalcitrant melasma. J Dermatol. 2007;34:25–30.

Freedman BM. Topical antioxidants enhance facial microdermabrasion. J of Dermatol Treat. 2009;20(2): 82–87.

Hexsel D, Mazzuco R, Dal'Forno T, et al. Microdermabrasion followed by a 5% retinoid acid chemical peel vs. a 5% retinoid acid chemical peel for the treatment of photoaging - a pilot study. J Cosmet Dermatol. 2005;4: 111–116.

Humphreys TR, Werth V, Dzubow L, et al. Treatment of photodamaged skin with trichloroacetic acid and topical tretinoin. J Am Acad Dermatol. 1996;34:638–644.

Lee WR, Shen SC, Kuo-Hsien W, et al. Lasers and microdermabrasion enhance and control topical delivery of vitamin C. J Invest Dermatol. 2003;121:1118–1125.

Lee WR, Tsai RY, Fang CL, et al. Microdermabrasion as a novel tool to enhance drug delivery via the skin: an animal study. Derm Surg. 2006;32:1013–1022.

Mark KA, Sparacio RM, Voigt A, et al. Objective and quantitative improvement of rosacea-associated erythema after intense pulsed light treatment. Derm Surg. 2003;29(6):600–604.

Papageorgiou P, Katasambas A, Chu A. Phototherapy with blue (415 nm) and red (660 nm) light in the treatment of acne vulgaris. Brit J Dermatol. 2000;142:973–978.

Pollock B, Turner D, Stringer MR, et al. Topical amiolaevulinic acid-photodynamic therapy for the treatment of acne vulgaris: study of clinical efficacy and mechanism of action. Brit J Dermatol. 2004;151:616–622.

Rendon M. Successful treatment of moderate to severe melasma with triple-combination cream and glycolic acid peels: a pilot study. Cutis. 2008;82(5):372–378.

Rendon MI, Effron C, Edison BL. The use of fillers and botulinum toxin type A in combination with superficial glycolic acid (alpha-hydroxy acid) peels: optimizing injection therapy with the skin-smoothing properties of peels. Cutis. 2007;79:9–12.

Sarkar R, Kaur C, Bhalla M, et al. The combination of glycolic acid peels with a topical regimen in the treatment of melasma in dark-skinned patients: a comparative study. Dermatol Surg. 2002;28:828–832; discussion 32.

Small R, Hoang D, eds. A Practical Guide to Botulinum Toxin Procedures. Philadelphia, PA. Lippincott Williams & Wilkins. 2012:16–17.

Small R, Hoang D, eds. A Practical Guide to Dermal Filler Procedures. Philadelphia, PA. Lippincott Williams & Wilkins. 2012:16.

Small R, Hoang D. Combining Cosmetic Treatments. In: Usatine R, Pfenninger J, Stulberg D, and Small R, eds. Dermatologic and Cosmetic Procedures in Office Practice. Philadelphia, PA. Elsevier. 2011;377–381.

Soliman MM, Ramadan SA, Bassiouny DA, et al. Combined trichloroacetic acid peel and topical ascorbic acid versus trichloroacetic acid peel alone in the treatment of melasma: a comparative study. J Cosmet Dermatol. 2007;6:89–94.

Song JY, Kang HA, Kim MY, et al. Damage and recovery of skin barrier function after glycolic acid chemical peeling and crystal microdermabrasion. Derm Surg. 2004;30:390–394.

Wang SQ, Counters JT, Flor ME, et al. Treatment of inflammatory facial acne with the 1,450 nm diode laser alone versus microdermabrasion plus the 1,450 nm laser: a randomized, split-face trial. Derm Surg. 2006;32: 249–255.

Zhou Y, Banga AK. Enhanced delivery of cosmeceuticals by microdermabrasion. J Cosmet Dermatol. 2011;10: 179–184.

Product Safety

Ravita TD, Tanner RS, Ahearn DG, et al. Post-consumer use efficacies of preservatives in personal care and topical drug products: relationship to preservative category. J Ind Microbiol Biotechnol. 2009;36:35–38.

Ross G. A perspective on the safety of cosmetic products: a position paper of the American Council on Science and Health. Int J Toxicol. 2006;25:269–277.

Stewart L, McCall K, Highlander S, et al. What Are We Growing in Our Makeup? Cosmet Dermatol. 2011; 24(6)

Complications

Cernik C, Gallina K, Brodell RT. The treatment of herpes simplex infections: an evidence-based review. Arch Intern Med. 2008;168:1137–1144.

Davies MG, Briffa DV, Greaves MW. Systemic toxicity from topically applied salicylic acid. Brit Med J. 1979;1(6164):661.

Duffy DM. Avoiding complications. In: Rubin MG, ed. Chemical Peels. Procedures in Cosmetic Dermatology. Philadelphia, PA: Elsevier Inc. 2006;137–169.

Farris P, Rietschel R. An unusual response to microdermabrasion. Dermatol Surg. 2002;28:606–608.

Hirsch R, Stier M. Complications and Their Management in Cosmetic Dermatology. Dermatol Clin. 2009;27(4):507–520.

Monheit GD. Facial resurfacing may trigger the herpes simplex virus. Cosmet Dermatol. 1995;8:9–16.

Sadick NS. Overview of complications of nonsurgical facial rejuvenation procedures. Clin Plast Surg. 2001;28(1):163.

Note: Page number followed by f and t indicates figure and table respectively.